What Real Patients
and Clients Are Saying About
The Sugar Detox

"The Sugar Detox changed the way I think about food and opened my eyes to my full health potential."

—David A., television and movie producer

"The Sugar Detox helped reset my sweet tooth and provided me with great alternatives to satisfy my sugar cravings!"

—Mia R., actress and writer

"The Sugar Detox was what I needed to get back in the proper mind-set to be eating healthily and eating the right amount of food. After pregnancy and five months of breast-feeding, I had convinced myself that fruit juice was healthy and ice cream was a great way to get my daily calcium. So I needed a swift kick, and the Sugar Detox was it."

—J. R., editor

"This diet is fabulous. It is the first diet I have been able to stick to for more than a week. I was not hungry at all, and the weight started coming off immediately. It was a major life change for me. I typically eat whatever I want, whenever I want it, including sugar, sweets, diet Coke, and alcohol. I found this not difficult at all, and I feel so good. I am more energetic, less lethargic, and just feel all around so much healthier. I am hoping this is the beginning of a major life change for me!"

—Stephanie L., consultant

"I've been trying to lose weight for years and find a good and healthy way of eating. The Sugar Detox has made me realize I do not need to drink diet soda or snack with unhealthy choices but allows me to make sensible decisions. I lost 11 pounds in one month, look great in my clothes, and never had so much energy."

—H. A., executive

"The Sugar Detox is not for the faint of heart—especially if you have a sweet tooth! Personally, I could eat dessert three times a day. So, the first three days were a serious challenge. My results, however, made it all worth it. My goal was simply to see if I could stick to the plan and limit my sugar intake. I was shocked that such a relatively minor adjustment in my eating habits made such a tremendous impact. I lost 7 pounds in ten days and found I had a clearer complexion. The plan made me realize just how much sugar I was routinely ingesting without even realizing it. Having modified the way I eat, I have been able to cut out those wasted sugars and truly enjoy the sweetness of a well-earned piece of dark chocolate."

—Stephanie F., attorney

"The Sugar Detox provided me with guidelines for sensible and healthy eating. I never once felt hungry on this diet. I lost over 6 pounds. It is so nice to be able to fit into clothes I have not worn since before I was pregnant with my daughter."

—Stacy, stay-at-home mom

"The diet worked miracles for my skin and overall mood. I didn't realize that sugar caused my skin to be irritated and itchy. Also, my mood was more level throughout the day, with not as many highs and lows. I'm very happy with the weight loss results as well!"

—Jennifer S., stay-at-home mom

"I lost 10 pounds in a month, feel good, am less tired, and couldn't be happier. What is most interesting, though, is that I used to get occasional hypoglycemic blood sugar drops and feel like I was going to pass out if I didn't eat something immediately to raise my blood sugar. But since I have been eating the Sugar Detox way, I haven't experienced that feeling even once—no instant rush of having to eat something, no postmeal crashes. It's as though my system kind of smoothed itself out. I definitely intend to keep eating this way."

—M. G., attorney

"The Sugar Detox awakened my senses. I have a newfound appreciation for how food should smell and taste and how good my body feels when I'm eating well."

—M. Z. G., product manager

"After a twenty-five-year career as a pastry chef, the Sugar Detox was the perfect antidote. It gently eased me into a healthier lifestyle—a lifestyle that was easy to adapt to after a lifetime of eating so much sugar and fats. I feel as if I'm ten years younger in just a month."

—Heather C.

"I never thought that I could rejuvenate myself by changing my diet. I have spent a fortune on products, procedures, and personal trainers but seem to have been missing the most important piece of the puzzle. The Sugar Detox helped me lose weight and the amazing thing is that my skin looks better than ever. Good-bye sugar, hello to a younger looking me."

—L. C., working mom

THE Sugar DETOX

Lose Weight, Feel Great, and Look Years Younger

Brooke Alpert and **Patricia Farris**
MS, RD, CDN   MD, FAAD

Da Capo
LIFE
LONG

A Member of the Perseus Books Group

Editorial production by Lori Hobkirk at the Book Factory
Set in 11.5 point Fairfield by the Perseus Books Group

Cataloging-in-Publication data for this book is available from
the Library of Congress.

First Da Capo Press edition 2013
ISBN: 978-0-7382-1641-6

Published by Da Capo Press
A Member of the Perseus Books Group
www.dacapopress.com

Note: the information in this book is true and complete to
the best of our knowledge. This book is intended only as an informative
guide for those wishing to know more about health issues. In no way is
this book intended to replace, countermand, or conflict with the advice
given to you by your own physician. The ultimate decision concerning care
should be made between you and your doctor. We strongly recommend you
follow his or her advice. Information in this book is general and is offered
with no guarantees on the part of the authors or Da Capo Press.
The authors and publisher disclaim all liability in connection with
the use of this book. The names and identifying details of people
associated with events described in this book have been changed.
Any similarity to actual persons is coincidental.

Da Capo Press books are available at special discounts for bulk purchases
in the U.S. by corporations, institutions, and other organizations.
For more information, please contact the Special Markets Department
at the Perseus Books Group, 2300 Chestnut Street, Suite 200,
Philadelphia, PA, 19103, or call (800) 810-4145, ext. 5000,
or e-mail special.markets@perseusbooks.com.

10 9 8 7 6 5 4 3 2 1

For our families, clients, and patients

CONTENTS

v

QUIZ
Are You a Sugar Addict?

1. Does eating sweets make you feel better if you're in a bad mood?
   A. Always
   B. Sometimes
   C. Never

2. Does eating starchy carbs (bread, cereal, pasta, potatoes, etc.) make you feel better if you're in a bad mood?
   A. Always
   B. Sometimes
   C. Never

3. Do you ever feel guilty about the amount of starchy carbs or sweets you consume?
   A. Always
   B. Sometimes
   C. Never

4. Have you ever tried to cut back on the amount of sugar you eat?
   A. Always
   B. Sometimes
   C. Never

5. Have you ever tried and failed to cut back on carbs?
   A. Always
   B. Sometimes
   C. Never

6. Are you unable to celebrate a birthday or other event without eating something sweet?
   A. Always
   B. Sometimes
   C. Never

7. Do you ever hide or deny the sweets you eat?
   A. Always
   B. Sometimes
   C. Never

8. Do you think about sugar or dessert even if you're not hungry?
   A. Always
   B. Sometimes
   C. Never

9. Can you not get through the day without sugar in your coffee, a soft drink, or some type of energy drink?
   A. Always
   B. Sometimes
   C. Never

10. Do you crash at 3 p.m. every day and look for something sweet to eat or drink to help?
    A. Always
    B. Sometimes
    C. Never

Now tally up your answers. How did you respond?

Mostly As	**Houston, we have a problem**—you're an addict. Off to rehab with our 3-Day Sugar Fix.
Mostly Bs	**You're middling here,** but there's plenty of room for improvement. Let's get you going!
Mostly Cs	**You rarely crave sugar**—great; now we can work on getting you to look and feel your best!

INTRODUCTION

Before we start, we're going to ask you to do something simple: Picture one of those 5-pound bags of sugar, the kind you find in your average grocery store. Got it? Now picture fifteen of them. Hang on to that image—we'll get back to it in a minute.

Ah, sugar—the sweet stuff we dash (or dump) in our coffee, sprinkle on our oatmeal, and caramelize on our crème brûlée. In this book, we're not just talking about the sweeteners we know we add to our foods to give it a little kick. We're also talking about all the hidden sugars—the ones you may not know about—that are in many of the most popular foods we consume. In fact, sugar consumption is at an all-time high, and it's making us unhealthy—so much so that a group of scientists from the University of California at San Francisco have recently recommended that the use of sugar be regulated the same way alcohol and tobacco are in the United States. Yep, sugar as a controlled substance!

Some people might find the government monitoring of sugar a bit much, but here's the scoop: A diet high in sugar, such as the one found right here in the USA, leads to everything from weight gain to heart disease and even type 2 diabetes. The Centers for Disease Control has projected that one in three Americans will have diabetes by 2050. The vast majority of these cases could probably be prevented if we just kept our weight under control, exercised more—and lowered our consumption of sugar.

Remember those fifteen bags of sugar you visualized? That's how much sugar the average American consumes each year. More than 70 pounds of it. And diabetes isn't the only problem caused by our over-consumption of sugar. Diets high in sugar also increase the risk for atherosclerosis, heart disease, Alzheimer's disease, and even cataracts. We'll get into the exact science a bit more later, but basically this is because sugars left unchecked in the bloodstream have to go somewhere, so they grab on to protein molecules throughout the body. These protein-sugar complexes, called advanced glycation end products, or AGEs, can be found in virtually all organ systems. AGEs trigger massive inflammation in the body, causing further tissue damage—and premature aging. So suffice it to say that these nasty little sugarcoated proteins are not our friends.

AGEs are unfortunately very aptly named: The collagen and elastin molecules that help your face defy gravity are extremely susceptible to being attacked by sugar. When these molecules are turned into AGEs, their soft and supple fibers become more rigid and can no longer do the heavy lifting needed to keep things in place. This whole sugary mess leaves skin saggy, baggy, and wrinkled.

In short, sugar is compromising our health, making us fat, lazy, and ugly. Maybe you've picked up this book because you're tired of feeling tired all the time, or maybe you've been diagnosed with a chronic condition that requires you to change your eating habits and lose weight. Regardless of your reason, our Sugar Detox program will help you become healthier, leaner, and, yes, younger looking. It has been designed specifically to stop sugar cravings and target and eliminate foods that cause weight gain, fatigue, and premature aging, while replacing them with foods that will give you energy, help you lose weight, and make you look younger. What's not to love?

Your Detoxing Dynamic Duo

What's unique about the Sugar Detox is that you're getting the combined expertise of a nutritionist and dermatologist. Every day, both of us see women complaining of weight gain, premature aging, and lack of energy. We created the Sugar Detox to help our patients reach their goals. It is a unique multidiscipline approach that will allow you to look and feel better from the inside out and the outside in.

Brooke R. Alpert, MS, RD, CDN, is the founder of B Nutritious, a private nutrition counseling practice in New York City. Brooke and her team at B Nutritious have been working with hundreds of women, men, and teenagers over the years to help change their diet to achieve weight loss, boost energy levels, and benefit overall health and wellness. It wasn't long into her practice that Brooke realized that sugar was the key player in how her patients felt. By reducing the amount of sugar they were eating and eliminating artificial sugars from their diet, Brooke's patients were able to get results so much quicker for losing weight, feeling more energized, and seeing their skin start to change. Now, all Brooke's patients follow a low-sugar diet and are incredibly successful with their weight loss and nutritional goals.

Dr. Patricia Farris is a board-certified dermatologist, clinical assistant professor at Tulane University, and internationally recognized expert on the treatment of aging skin. Dr. Farris became interested in the relationship between nutrition and aging when she realized that some of her patients seeking cosmetic procedures were aged way beyond their years. She noticed that many of these patients did not have the usual signs and symptoms of sun damage, but their skin was still excessively wrinkled with a marked loss in elasticity. The culprits? Poor nutrition and excessive sugar consumption. Frustrated by those who were willing to pay big bucks for such quick fixes as laser treatments and chemical peels but unwilling to make the diet and lifestyle changes that were really required to make them look and feel younger, she teamed up with Brooke to create an easy diet program that would help her patients achieve their goals. Dr. Farris now routinely recommends the Sugar Detox diet as part of a comprehensive treatment plan for patients who suffer from premature aging, acne, and other skin conditions. By combining our expertise for you, *The Sugar Detox* is a sure-fire way to help you look and feel your absolute best. Throughout the book, we share stories from our practices and patients—people just like you whom we've helped to break free from sugar to be healthier, happier— and who look amazing!

The Key to Inside-Out and Outside-In Health

We've developed a 3-Day Sugar Fix that will help you break free immediately from your sugar dependence. Sugar truly is addictive: Your body reacts to it like a drug and craves it constantly. What we're asking you to do is to quit—cold turkey. We won't lie: These three days are tough, but with every bite and sip you will start to feel better and be on the road to a healthier, more beautiful life. The 3-Day Sugar Fix program starts right after this introduction, so get ready to start healthy living now. We want you to see and feel the results you want as quickly as possible, and so although the rest of the book will certainly help you stick to a committed plan (and will give you all the necessary science and rationale for why sugar is so bad and what it really does to your body), we prefer that you get to work on the program right away, and continue reading as you undergo the 3-Day Sugar Fix.

We want you to feel positive about this diet instead of deprived, so after the 3-Day Sugar Fix, you'll find chapters that explain what foods you should be eating on a regular basis, why they are good for you, and how even your favorite foods (chocolate, cheese, wine, and more) can actually be beneficial for you. Then we move on to the foods to avoid, how to eat throughout the day, how to care for your skin, and how to tone up with an exercise program that's specifically created to work in tandem with the diet plan. At the end of the book are recipes we created with our amazing chef, Jason Brown, which are delicious, satisfying, and all Sugar Detox approved!

The diet is broken up into four weeks and each week is slightly different. It's hardest in the beginning, but the good news is that each week, we gradually add some more options for you choose from. We want you to be as prepared as possible before starting out, so that you'll have an easier time staying on the plan. To that end, we include meal plans, 3-day and weekly approved-food lists, plus suggestions for the best meals to choose when dining out. Always take a look at the food lists for each week and make sure you're fully stocked at home, so you have less to worry about when that week starts. By the end of the four weeks, you will have completed an amazing physical transformation and will feel as if you can conquer the world!

Throughout the book, you'll hear from our patients and clients—women and men just like you who've kicked their sugar habits and now embrace a healthier lifestyle and years-younger looks. You'll also find some prescriptions throughout—Rx's that help you along the way.

So that's the plan. We hope you're excited for the immediate and lifelong changes that you're about to make starting right away with the 3-Day Sugar Fix. Within no time at all, you'll be feeling and looking better than ever and know that you're making a healthy commitment to yourself and your body. We're in this with you!

What You Need to Know Before Starting the Sugar Detox

- If you are a diabetic or have any type of blood sugar problem including insulin resistance, it is essential to consult your physician before starting any type of diet program, including the Sugar Detox.
- If you are taking insulin or any other medication to control blood sugar and start a low sugar diet such as the Sugar Detox, consult your physician as you will probably require less than your current dose of medication.
- The Sugar Detox diet may not be appropriate for those who engage in extreme exercise programs, such as long-distance running, cycling, or other intense cardiovascular workouts.
- During the 3-Day Sugar Fix you may experience fatigue, fogginess, headaches, and intense cravings as you detox off sugar. In most cases these symptoms will resolve as you continue the program but should they persist we suggest you discontinue and consult your physician.

Part One

THE Sugar-Free Prescription

1

Rx 1: The 3-Day Sugar Fix

Three days without sugar? You may be thinking to yourself that that's going to be pretty hard. And we won't lie to you—it can be difficult. But it's just three days. Think of what three days are in proportion to the rest of your life—and how these three days in particular will help you commit to health and radiance that can last a lifetime!

Our 3-Day Sugar Fix is simple: no dairy, no fruit aside from lemon or lime, no wheat or starches, and no added sugars. As you'll soon see, the plan is also pretty basic; we keep the list of approved foods the same across the three days to make your detox as clear and simple as possible: We wanted to give you some freedom, so if you prefer your breakfast eggs poached, great! If you want to scramble them with veggies, that's great, too. We just ask that you adhere to this list of foods . . . but within those parameters, feel free to get creative!

Here are the guidelines for all three days (yes, they really are that simple).

3-Day Sugar Fix Approved Foods
- 1 cup of unsweetened black coffee per day
- Unsweetened green and/or herbal tea, in unlimited amounts
- Minimum 64 ounces of water (sodium-free sparkling water or club soda is okay) daily

- Protein: lean red meat, pork, chicken, turkey, fish, shellfish, eggs, tofu, or legumes (see box below for vegetarian/vegan options; see list of approved proteins on page 7)
- Veggies: approved veggies (see page 7) in unlimited amounts
- Fruits: lemon or lime, for drinks or cooking
- Nuts: a 1-ounce serving of nuts (see page 7) may be eaten up to twice daily as a snack.
- Condiments and cooking oil: red wine vinegar, balsamic vinegar, or apple cider vinegar; and olive oil, coconut oil, or butter for cooking
- Herbs and spices: unlimited amounts

No-No's
- Artificial sweeteners of any kind—and that includes diet drinks
- Alcohol
- Dairy (except a little butter for cooking)
- Wheat or other starches, such as pasta, cereal, bread, rice, or quinoa
- Added sugar of any kind
- Fruit (except lemon or lime for drinks or cooking)

Cooking Techniques
- Sauté
- Stir-fry
- Poach
- Steam
- Boil

Remember to use only the oils on the approved list!

Vegetarians and Vegans

The Sugar Detox can be followed by both vegetarians and vegans. Tofu can replace any meat or egg product for any meal. Legumes, such as beans, can also be your protein substitute; just watch your portion sizes. Unsweetened almond, coconut, or soy milk, or yogurt, can be used as a dairy substitute. Just read the ingredients to make sure no sugars, such as evaporated cane syrup, are listed.

Daily MENUS

Every day, you will start with a healthy breakfast, eat a satisfying lunch, and enjoy a delicious dinner—and you have our blessing to snack between meals! See Chapter 13 or Recipe Index (page 257) for the recipes for asterisked items.

The Basic Meal Plan

BREAKFAST: three eggs, any style (include herbs and approved vegetables, if desired), cooked with only approved oils

SNACK: 1 ounce of nuts

LUNCH: up to 6 ounces of chicken, turkey, fish, shellfish, or tofu, plus a small salad with any of these vegetable options: arugula, asparagus, avocado, bok choy, broccoli, Brussels sprouts, cabbage (Chinese, red, or green), cauliflower, celery, cucumbers, kale, lettuce (romaine, red leaf, or green leaf), mushrooms, peppers (bell or hot peppers), spinach, or zucchini

SNACK: sliced peppers with hummus

DINNER: chicken, turkey, fish, shellfish, or tofu (up to 8 ounces) and a large portion of steamed mixed approved vegetables

Day 1

BREAKFAST: three scrambled eggs with pinch of dried rosemary, unsweetened green tea with lemon, a large glass of water with lime

SNACK: Sweetish Nuts*, unsweetened cinnamon tea

LUNCH: 6 ounces of Poached Chicken Breasts* on top of mixed baby greens and ½ sliced avocado with herbs, olive oil, and red wine vinegar

SNACK: sliced red and green bell peppers with 2 tablespoons of Spinach Hummus*, a large glass of water with lime

DINNER: ½ cup of edamame, salmon with stir-fried broccoli and mushrooms

Day 2

BREAKFAST: 3 eggs scrambled with sautéed spinach

SNACK: ½ ounce of roasted almonds, unsweetened iced green tea with lemon

LUNCH: Tuna Niçoise: canned tuna or a sautéed fresh tuna steak over a bed of mixed greens, one hard-boiled egg sliced, and steamed haricots verts, dressed with Sugar Detox Vinaigrette*

SNACK: sliced peppers with hummus

DINNER: rosemary pork tenderloin, sautéed Brussels sprouts and mushrooms seasoned with salt, pepper and fresh garlic, chopped romaine salad with avocado dressed with lemon and extra virgin olive oil.

Day 3

BREAKFAST: three-egg omelet with shrimp, sautéed spinach and tarragon

SNACK: 1 oz. cashews

LUNCH: grilled turkey burger with sliced heirloom tomatoes, lettuce, and sautéed mushrooms, plus kale chips

SNACK: sliced peppers with hummus

DINNER: baked tilapia over bok choy and cherry tomatoes, plus mixed greens with Sugar Detox Vinaigrette*

The 3-Day Sugar Fix Shopping List

Along with being your go-to shopping list for the first three days of the Sugar Detox, this list forms the basis of the following four weeks' approved foods (we'll get into that in more detail in Chapter 8). Where applicable, your serving size per meal is given in parentheses, to help you plan your grocery shopping.

Proteins

Eggs (3)
Lean red meat (6 ounces)
Pork (6 ounces)
Chicken (6 ounces)
Turkey (6 ounces)

Fish (6 ounces)
Shellfish (6 ounces)
Tofu (6 ounces)
Legumes (lentils, beans,
    edamame, peas) (½ cup)

Vegetables

UNLIMITED EXCEPT FOR AVOCADO.

Arugula
Asparagus
Avocado (also counted as a
    fat; ½ max per day)
Bok choy
Broccoli
Brussels sprouts
Cabbage (Chinese, red, or
    green)
Cauliflower

Celery
Cucumbers
Kale
Lettuce (romaine lettuce,
    red leaf, green leaf)
Mushrooms
Peppers (bell or hot peppers)
Spinach
Zucchini

Fruit

Lemon or lime

Nuts and Seeds

NUTS MAY BE ROASTED OR RAW, AND SHOULD IDEALLY BE UN-SALTED: 1 OUNCE PER SERVING. (FOR MORE INFORMATION ABOUT FLAX-, CHIA, AND HEMP SEEDS, SEE THE BOX ON PAGE 72.)

Almonds
Cashews
Chia seeds
Flaxseeds
Hemp seeds

Macadamia
Peanuts
Pecans
Pistachios
Walnuts

Fats and Oils

Butter (1 tablespoon)
Coconut oil (1 tablespoon)
Olive oil (1 tablespoon)
Olives (10 olives)

Condiments

Balsamic vinegar
Apple cider vinegar
Red wine vinegar

Herbs/Spices

ALL SPICES ARE GREAT, ESPECIALLY THOSE LISTED HERE.

YOU'LL NOTICE THAT SALT ISN'T ON THIS LIST; WE'D PREFER YOU TRY SOME NEW FLAVORS. SALT IS OKAY TO USE ON OUR WEEK-BY-WEEK SUGAR DETOX PLAN BUT SHOULD BE USED IN MODERATION.

Ginger
Allspice
Cinnamon
Cloves
Marjoram

Rosemary
Sage
Tarragon
Turmeric

Beverages

ENJOY THESE IN UNLIMITED QUANTITIES.

Water
Sodium-free club soda or sparkling water
Coffee (unsweetened, black)
Green tea (unsweetened)
Black tea (unsweetened)
Herbal tea (unsweetened)

After seeing the 3-Day Sugar Fix meal plan and shopping list, you might think that the Sugar Detox is just another low-carb diet. It's true that the 3-Day Sugar Fix doesn't allow you any bread, rice, or pasta, but that is because starchy carbohydrates are a major contributor to sugar addiction (more on this in a minute). We replace them with good carbohydrates that are full of fiber, come from vegetables, and can actually help lower your blood sugar. You may also have noticed that we're not offering a low-carbohydrate diet where you can eat tons of fatty protein, such as bacon and steak. Instead, we give you lean, low-fat protein options and plenty of vegetables that will fill you up without weighing you down and clogging your arteries.

Sweet **Talk**

BA says:

"If drinking coffee without milk and sugar seems impossible, try it iced!"

2

Rx 2: The 3-Day Skin Fix

The first three days of the Sugar Detox are the most difficult as you begin to kick the sugar habit. We know our intensive 3-Day Sugar Fix can be trying, so on these days we are going to pamper you with a regimen that includes soothing, spalike treatments that can be done in the comfort of your own home. These treatments have been selected because they contain natural ingredients and have therapeutic benefits that improve skin health and beauty.

Day 1: Balance Your Skin with a Sea Mud Mask

As you'll discover in later chapters, we are high on the natural benefits of the sea. Sea mud is composed of nineteen different minerals, including the skin savers magnesium, zinc, and sulfur. The soil portion of sea mud is composed of organic matter called humus and has natural healing properties. Not only is sea mud used to restore the pH balance of the skin and help maintain skin hydration, it also increases circulation and has natural anti-aging properties. Sea mud cleanses the skin, removes surface oils, and discards dead skin cells. Sea mud has natural antibacterial ingredients, so masks made with it are helpful for those with acne. With all these benefits how could we not suggest that you enjoy a sea mud mask as part of the 3-Day Skin Fix?

Sea mud can be purchased in its natural form. Make certain to buy sea mud that can be used on the face, as many products are labeled for body only. Wash your face with a gentle cleanser and then apply a thin coat of the mud mask to your entire face, avoiding sensitive areas, such as the skin just below your eyes and your eyelids. The mud will turn a lighter color as it dries. As the mask dries, it gently lifts away dead skin cells, unwanted surface oils and helps repair and revitalize the skin. It should be removed by rinsing with warm water once the process is complete. Your skin may feel tight after the mask is removed, so feel free to apply a light moisturizer if your face is dry. It is always best to apply a small amount of the mask to your neck before using it on more tender facial skin.

Although purists prefer the real stuff, you may be better served to try a ready-prepared sea mud mask. These masks contain sea mud, are easy to apply, and are generally less drying. Many commercially available products are embellished with such beneficial ingredients as antioxidants, soothing aloe vera, jojoba, and essential oils. Each mask will provide guidance as to what skin type it is suited for and how long it should be left on the skin. And don't forget that your face isn't the only place where you can use sea mud products. Body wraps with sea mud are touted for exfoliating, toning, and improving cellulite. So why not get a little dirty?

Day 2: Ancient Beauty Bath

There is nothing more relaxing than a long, warm, soaking bath. This is why on Day 2 we suggest you enjoy one of the oldest therapeutic remedies: bathing in salts from the sea. You can choose from Black Sea salt, French sea salt, Italian sea salt, Hawaiian sea salt and Dead Sea salt just to name a few. It's important to understand we are not talking about using gourmet sea salt in your bath. Salts processed for bathing are specially prepared and come in different sizes, shapes, and colors. Adding sea salt to your bath can stimulate circulation, ease muscle aches and pains, and soothe the body. One of our favorites is Dead Sea salt because of its unique composition and medicinal properties. The healing power of Dead Sea salt is due to its high concentration of magnesium and other minerals including sodium, potassium, and calcium. Magnesium salts are known to improve skin hydration, reduce redness and inflamation. Studies have confirmed the skin-smoothing benefits of Dead Sea salt, making it a favorite in salons and spas that offer total body rejuvenation. Don't just take it from us; for years, dermatologists have recommended Dead Sea salt soaks to patients with such inflammatory skin disorders as psoriasis and eczema. Even Cleopatra recognized the rejuvenating value of the Dead Sea and made regular trips to the region to enjoy its benefits! So go ahead and treat yourself like royalty: Enjoy a long soaking bath in Dead Sea salt.

To enhance the experience, add a couple of drops of your favorite essential oil to your bath. As you are filling the tub, we suggest you dry brush your entire body. Dry brushing helps improve circulation and removes fluids and swelling from the tissues by improving lymphatic drainage. It will make your skin feel smoother immediately and is a great way to remove puffiness. Dry brushing also helps enhance the therapeutic benefits of the sea salt bath.

Using a natural-bristle brush or mitt, run the brush across your skin in short, brisk stokes, using an upward motion. Start at the soles of your feet, moving up your legs, brushing upward toward your heart. When you have completed your legs, brush your entire body upward, then repeat the process starting at the tips of your fingers, brushing upward along your arms. Once you have completed your body brushing, add a half-cup of sea salt to your bath. Turn off your cell phone, put on some relaxing music, and enjoy one of the oldest therapeutic soaks known to man.

Day 3: Fight Back with Supercharged Antioxidants

Okay, you're in the home stretch and you've made it to Day 3 of the Sugar Fix. Today's regime will neutralize free radicals, protect your skin, and treat troubled areas, such as puffy under-eye bags. For your face, we suggest a moisturizing antioxidant mask. There are plenty to choose from; some of our favorites are those that contain blueberry, green tea, black tea, rosemary extract, resveratrol, or algae extract. You may find products containing more than one antioxidant ingredient, so we say, the more the merrier. Choose a mask that is cream based and will hydrate your skin while fighting free radicals.

If you enjoy do-it-yourself projects, try processing in a blender ½ cup of full-fat or 2% Greek yogurt, 1 tablespoon of ground old-fashioned rolled oats (grind to a fine powder in a coffee or spice grinder; do not use instant oats), 1 tablespoon of honey, and a handful of crushed blueberries. The yogurt contains exfoliating lactic acid, oatmeal is a natural anti-inflammatory, honey has healing properties and acts as a natural moisturizer, and the blueberries contain powerful antioxidants. Apply a thin layer of the mixture to your face and let it work its magic. This mask should be left on for ten minutes and washed off with warm water.

For troubled areas such as the under eye, might we suggest you try a simple home remedy of green tea compresses to reduce puffiness. We'll be preaching about the benefits of green tea throughout the book, but who knew that this simple home brew of green tea could be used to improve one of the most pesky skin problems? Just prepare a quart of green tea, using two tea bags. Let it cool and then refrigerate until chilled. Soak cotton balls in the tea, lean back, and gently apply the cotton as a compress on the areas around your eyes for five to ten minutes. This treatment will leave your skin glowing—without any impact on your wallet!

3-Day Skin Fix Recommended Products

Sea Mud/Sea Mud Masks

Borghese Fango Active Mud Face and Body. This mud, sourced from Tuscany's volcanic hills, can be used as a facial mask or body treatment.

Adovia Purifying Mud Mask. This mask contains Dead Sea minerals and soothing aloe vera and vitamin C. They also offer Adovia 100 percent pure Dead Sea mud.

Erno Laszlo Sea Mud Exfoliating Mask. This mask absorbs oils and gently exfoliates dead skin cells. Best for normal to oily skin.

Honeymark's Mud Mask. This unique combination of Dead Sea mud and Manuka Honey from New Zealand revitalizes the skin and restores moisture.

Keihl's White Clay Mask. White clay from the mouth of the Amazon River combined with aloe vera and oatmeal.

SkinCeuticals Clarifying Clay Mask. A combination of clay, aloe vera, chamomile, phloretin, and a blend of alpha hydroxy acids make this mask great for all skin types.

Sea Salts

San Francisco Bath Salt Company offers a variety of bath sea salts, including Pacific, European, and Dead Sea salt.

SaltWorks. If you are looking for unique sea salts such as Himalayan and Hawaiian Red, this is a great resource. They also offer Atlantic, European, and Dead Sea salt.

Antioxidant Masks

MD Formulations Moisture Defense Antioxidant Treatment Masque. Designed as a super-hydration treatment, this mask serves up a healthy dose of natural antioxidants, including vitamin E, green tea extract, chamomille extract, and calming licorice extract.

Apivita Express Beauty Revitalizing Mask with Pomegranate. Infused with antioxidant-rich pomegranate and green tea, this mask contains natural moisturizers including honey, olive oil, and vitamins.

Origins Drink Up 10-Minute Mask to Quench Skin's Thirst. Contains algae extract and apricot oil.

Clinique Moisture Surge Mask. Algae extract and mango seed butter, a dynamic duo for this moisturizing mask.

Jan Marini Age Intervention Regeneration Mask. Made with resveratrol, peptides, glycolic acid, and antioxidants (green tea, white tea, pomegranate extract).

Koh Gen Do Oriental Plants Deep Moisture Mask. Combines red, green, and brown algae extract; vitamin E; and jojoba oil. This mask is left on overnight to give you a beauty treatment while you sleep.

Caudalie Masque-Crème Hydrant. This creamy mask boasts potent antioxidants derived from grapes.

Boscia Intensifying Moisture Pack +. Combining the best of both worlds this mask includes plant and algae extract plus beta carotene.

Part **Two**

Everything You Need to Know About the **Sugar Detox**

The Sweet Dilemma

We've talked a little bit about the science behind sugar and why it's so bad for us. But did you know that there are sugars hidden in a great number of packaged foods? Take the following Sugar IQ Quiz to get a sense of some of the sneakier aspects of the sweet stuff.

Test Your Sugar IQ

1. Which one contains more sugar?
   - A. Snapple Lemon Tea (16-ounce bottle)
   - B. Coca Cola (12-ounce can)
   - C. Starbucks Vanilla Latte (Tall, 12 fluid ounces)

2. Acne is caused by
   - A. Genetics
   - B. Hormonal changes
   - C. Stress
   - D. Poor diet
   - E. All of the above

3. Wrinkles are most affected by
   - A. Sun damage
   - B. Smoking
   - C. Poor fluid status
   - D. Poor diet high in sugar
   - E. All of the above

4. The average American consumes _____ of added sugar each day.
   - A. 31 teaspoons
   - B. 18 teaspoons
   - C. 10 teaspoons
   - D. 25 teaspoons

5. True or false? Humans naturally prefer the taste of sugar from birth.

6. True or false? Sugar toxicity causes liver damage.

7. True or false? Sugar substitutes help control weight gain.

8. Which of these foods is hiding the most sugar per ½ cup serving?
   - A. Tomato sauce
   - B. Salsa
   - C. Tomato soup

9. What's the difference in calories from sugar between a "fun size" and regular Snickers bar?
   - A. 13
   - B. 24
   - C. 49
   - D. 78

10. Reduced-fat packaged foods often have
   - A. Less sugar than the full-fat version
   - B. More sugar than the full-fat version
   - C. The same amount of sugar as the full-fat version

11. The difference in sugar between a 12-ounce glass of orange juice and an orange is
   - A. 8 g
   - B. 13 g
   - C. 16 g

12. True or false? Eating too much sugar causes wrinkles.

13. True or false? Natural sugars, such as honey, have less of an effect on the body than refined sugar does.

14. True or false? Natural sugars, such as honey, have fewer calories than refined sugar.

15. True or false? People with high blood sugar generally look older.

Answers: 1. B; 2. E; 3. E; 4. A; 5. True; 6. True; 7. False; 8. A; 9. D; 10. B; 11. C; 12. True; 13. False; 14. False; 15. True.

How many answers did you get right?

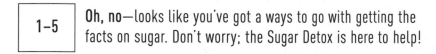

Oh, no—looks like you've got a ways to go with getting the facts on sugar. Don't worry; the Sugar Detox is here to help!

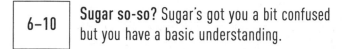

Sugar so-so? Sugar's got you a bit confused but you have a basic understanding.

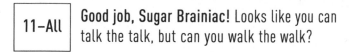

Good job, Sugar Brainiac! Looks like you can talk the talk, but can you walk the walk?

How'd you do? These facts are just the tip of the iceberg of why both the sugar you add and the sugar that's been added for you are so bad for your health. Here's some more info on how dastardly that sweet stuff actually is.

Sugar in Disguise

Obesity, heart disease, and diabetes are all on the rise. According to a study published in the *Journal of the American Medical Association*, more than 35 percent of all American adults were clinically obese in 2010—a twofold increase in the rate of obesity, compared to Americans in the 1960s. Several studies have found a correlation in the rise of obesity with an increase in sugar consumption. Not only that, the Centers for Disease Control and Prevention (CDC) reports that in the United States about 1.9 million people aged twenty years or older were newly diagnosed with diabetes in 2010, and 27.1 million people are currently diagnosed with heart disease.

So what's changed in the last fifty years, besides our waistline and medical bills? The United States Department of Agriculture (USDA) found that Americans are eating 39 percent more sugar than they were fifty years ago. The average person is now eating 32 teaspoonfuls of added sugars per day—well over the recommended number of no more than 10 teaspoons per day (the amount of sugar in one 12-ounce soda).

The USDA also found that Americans' average daily calorie intake has increased by almost 25 percent. A huge amount of that increase was found to come from diets full of refined grain products, aside from added sugars. In fact, Americans are eating an average of eleven servings of grains per day—mostly refined grains with little to no fiber. What's the big deal? Simply put, refined grains—which include white rice, white flour, and also many cereals, crackers, breads, and desserts—are basically sugar in disguise. During their processing, the nutrients and fiber are removed. It's the removal of fiber—the "refining"—that makes these grains so unhealthy. Fiber is good for you: It slows down the entire digestive process so that the absorption of sugar from grains is at a steadier pace; it also adds bulk to food, which leads to your feeling fuller sooner, which means you're more likely to eat less and therefore maintain a healthier weight.

There are two main types of fiber, soluble and insoluble. Soluble fiber attracts water and forms a gel inside the digestive system, delaying the emptying of your stomach and thereby allowing you to feel fuller longer. This gel puts up a barrier that acts like a roadblock to prevent cholesterol from being absorbed. Slower digestion also helps maintain stable blood sugar levels and can help with insulin sensitivity. In addition, soluble fiber helps lower LDL "bad" cholesterol—a heart-healthy plus right there! Insoluble fiber, on the other hand, is the kind of fiber that helps pass bulk through your digestive system and keeps your system moving efficiently. Both types of fiber are imperative to a healthy life and are important on the Sugar Detox plan. Consuming a large amount of refined grains, which lack this vital element of fiber, is likely one major reason why people in the United States are gaining weight rapidly and being diagnosed with all of these chronic diseases.

Sugar—The Fourth Food Group?

Let's break this down. There are three main food groups: proteins, fats, and carbohydrates. We know that each of these food groups has a unique function in the body and that all of them are necessary for good health.

Proteins are found in all animal products, such as meat, eggs, poultry, and dairy, as well as in nuts and legumes. Proteins are made up of smaller molecules called amino acids that serve as building blocks for bone, muscle, hair, skin, and nails. Amino acids can also be turned into enzymes, hormones, and antibodies that are necessary to keep your body healthy. Protein is important in your diet, as it provides your body with essential amino acids that it cannot synthesize.

Fats, like proteins, are also essential. Fats are found in oils, nuts, seeds, and certain types of fish. Fats are used as lubricants in the body and provide insulation for vital organs and from the cold. They can also be used to make steroid hormones and serve as carriers for fat-soluble vitamins. Omega-3 fatty acids are the standout essential fat that you need to get from your diet. They are responsible for keeping inflammation under control in the body, supporting heart health, lowering triglycerides and improving insulin resistance. Recent studies have also shown these essential fatty acids to be helpful for multiple other illnesses and conditions including depression, ADHD, Alzheimer's disease, and more. Of course, by now we have all gotten the message that there are good fats and bad fats, but rest assured, the Sugar Detox diet plan provides a healthy dose of only the good ones. (You'll find more on the benefits of healthy fats in Chapter 5.)

Carbohydrates are the main energy source for the body. Their primary function is to provide fuel for the brain, central nervous system, and muscles. Without carbohydrates, your body is basically like a car that's running out of gas. Your brain becomes foggy and you become tired, lacking the physical stamina you need to perform even the simplest task. This is why marathon runners, endurance athletes, and triathletes eat huge bowls of pasta or rice leading up to the night before a race. Athletes, who call this carbohydrate loading, use it to provide their body with the fuel it will need to sustain itself through the race. Now, much like fats, there are good carbs and bad ones; the main ways to separate the good from the bad are based on what kind of sugar they contain, how they are absorbed into the body, and how the body reacts to them.

Nancy had struggled with her weight since college. Now at forty-four years old, she was a solid 35 pounds overweight and not happy with herself. She'd tried every diet out there, from Weight Watchers to Atkins to master cleanses, but the weight would always come back as quickly as she lost it—and with some extra pounds added. When Brooke took a history of Nancy's eating habits, she found that Nancy was consuming large amounts of artificial sweeteners on a regular basis. She drank at least three diet sodas a day and ate artificially sweetened yogurts and desserts. When Brooke asked Nancy why she ate them, Nancy responded that they were "low in calories or points." When asked whether she had a sweet tooth, Nancy replied, "I don't eat much dessert." While Nancy may not be eating dessert regularly, she certainly was consuming a significant amount of unhealthy artificial sweeteners. Brooke weaned Nancy off her diet sodas and artificially sweetened desserts and slowly the weight started to come off. A few weeks later, Nancy was down 10 pounds and so was motivated to keep going. She couldn't believe how much her palate had changed, saying, "Who would have thought onions and almonds were so sweet!"

The Skinny on Carbs

Carbohydrates can be classified into two groups, complex or simple, based on their chemical structure. Complex carbohydrates are made up of long chains of sugars, whereas simple carbohydrates are much shorter chains.

Simple carbohydrates have just one or two sugars, and are easily digested in the small intestines, causing a quick spike in blood sugar once they enter the bloodstream. Simple carbohydrates are found in fruit (fructose), milk (galactose), table sugar (sucrose), and some vegetables and beer (maltose). While many simple carbohydrates are found in foods that are considered "good for you" such as dairy, fruits, and vegetables, they are also found in processed and refined foods, such as candy, soda, and syrups. When used in these latter products as sweeteners, simple sugars add calories without providing vitamins, minerals, or fiber to make them worth eating.

Complex carbohydrates, on the other hand, are made of three or more sugars and take far longer to digest. All complex carbohydrates are broken down by the body into glucose. They are found in legumes; starchy vegetables, such as sweet potatoes; and whole grains, such as those found in multigrain breads. These complex carbs contain vitamins, minerals, and most important, fiber. So while they still contain sugar, they are broken down more slowly than simple carbohydrates, causing less of a spike in blood sugar.

While you eat, the primary goal of your body is to break down the food into small molecules and then absorb them. The real issues here are how quickly the carbohydrate is broken down and absorbed, and whether it causes a rapid rise in blood sugar. The refining process, during which the bran and germ are stripped away from a whole grain, was developed to make grains finer and to give them a longer shelf life. Refined grains are lighter, fluffier, and easier to chew, but the downside is that they are stripped of all nutrients and fiber. Refined grains include white rice (which is refined brown rice), white bread, pasta, and the white flour found in most commercially baked goods. Because the refining process removes fiber, your body breaks down these carbohydrates far more quickly, causing a sugar blast in the bloodstream. On the other hand, unrefined whole grains, such as brown rice, quinoa, buckwheat, popcorn, and oatmeal are broken down more far more slowly. They also retain their nutritional value, providing a healthy dose of B-complex vitamins, iron, and other nutrients.

It is also important to understand that simple carbohydrates come in unrefined and refined versions, too. Fruits such as apples contain simple carbohydrates plus fiber, so they are considered to be unrefined, whereas fruit juices have no fiber and provide only refined simple carbohydrates. Ultimately, whole grains and whole fruits consumed in healthy portions are your best choice.

Why Sugar Is the Bad Guy

To understand why sugar is the bad guy, you need to understand how the body metabolizes sugars. Once sugar (glucose) is absorbed into the bloodstream, a hormone called insulin is triggered. Insulin is the regulator of sugar metabolism and determines how it is used in the body. Ideally, glucose in the bloodstream is taken up by cells and used as an energy source. Excess circulating glucose gets stored in the liver as glycogen, or ends up converting to fat. If the body is running low on glucose, the pancreas secretes another hormone called glucagon. When glucagon is released, it signals the liver to convert glycogen back to glucose, and the cells are happy again. Sounds so simple—too much glucose, you store it; not enough, you use your reserves. But for many of us, that's not always the case.

The Lows of the Sugar High

Because we are eating foods filled with added sugars, consuming too many refined carbohydrates, and drinking sugary drinks, while not eating healthy fats, protein, or enough fiber, we are sending our body into a sugar high. All that extra sugar that we're eating is flooding our bloodstream and sending constant alarms to our pancreas to release more insulin. Insulin tries to control the sugar situation by telling the liver to make more glycogen. Muscle also stores glycogen, but once these organs are full, the liver starts to turn excess sugar into triglycerides. This fat is stored in the liver and in fat cells throughout the body. Therefore, the more sugar we eat, the more insulin is released and the more fat we store. Insulin inhibits the breakdown of fat in fatty tissues, so when insulin is present, fat will get stored instead of burned.

Insulin plays "good cop" and "bad cop" in your body. It's the good guy when you eat something with sugar, because it jumps in to control the sugar riot in your bloodstream. Yet, it's also the bad guy because, while it's controlling the sugar situation, it is depositing fat in places where you don't want it, such as around your belly. The triglycerides produced

SWEET SUCCESS
Jessie

Jessie never had a weight problem before. She was always thin, even though she wasn't one for much exercise and never watched what she ate. While she always had a little tummy that bothered her, her main concern was her lack of energy. Jessie was known to her friends and family as "the Super Napper" because she could fall asleep anywhere, anytime, and was always in need of another nap. She came to Brooke looking to find a way to have more energy. During the initial session at B Nutritious, Brooke did a comprehensive history of her health background and of her eating habits. Jessie wasn't the epitome of health. Her tummy pooch was noticeable, her skin and hair lacked luster, and she had prominent dark circles under her eyes. What struck Brooke most was how much food this petite woman was eating. Jessie was consuming huge amounts of sugar without even realizing it: She started her day with a sugar-coated cereal, snacked on supposed health bars throughout the morning, had sandwiches and flavored yogurt for lunch, and ate pizza or pasta for dinner. She also drank a fair amount of alcohol, opting for sweet cocktails such as Cosmopolitans and Apple Martinis. Brooke immediately started Jessie on the Sugar Detox regimen and coached her through how to switch some of her old favorites to new and improved options. A week later, when Jessie came back into the office for her follow-up, Brooke was surprised by the immediate difference. Already the dark circles were gone from beneath Jessie's eyes and her tummy was noticeably flatter. Jessie, herself, was surprised that so much could change in one week. After completing the 31-day program, Jessie's stomach was completely flat for the first time in her life, her skin was the clearest it had ever been, and she had begun to actually enjoy exercise. The best part was that her family had to come up with a new nickname for her: They now call her the Energizer Bunny!

by the liver also spill out into the bloodstream, making you prone to clogged arteries and increasing your risk of heart attacks. In data just released from the Nurses' Health Study, one of the largest and longest-running studies of women's health, nurses whose diet had a higher sugar content experienced an almost twofold increased risk for heart disease.

The Skinny on Fat

All this weight gain and fat storage from all the excess sugar is more than just a size problem. Fat can be stored two ways: in subcutaneous tissues or internally. We've all seen subcutaneous fat in the form of a muffin top or thunder thighs; the far greater concern is internal fat.

Internal, or visceral, fat is deposited primarily around the abdominal organs, causing what known as the dreaded the beer belly or apple shape. What's even scarier is that there are people who look relatively thin on the outside, but because of sugar bingeing, they have tremendous amounts of fat on the inside. Being thin on the outside and fat on the inside can lure people into a sense of false security of not realizing just how unhealthy their high-sugar diet has made them. The medical profession now views visceral fat as the most dangerous kind, as it is associated with an increased risk of insulin resistance, heart disease, and certain cancers, including breast and colorectal.

Insulin resistance is when the body becomes almost numb to insulin and doesn't respond quickly or effectively to the hormone. This leads to an excess of sugar in the bloodstream. This in turn causes more ineffective insulin to be released, and so begins a vicious cycle. While there is definitely a genetic predisposition in those who develop insulin resistance, obesity and lack of exercise are major contributing factors. People with insulin resistance do not realize that they are sick because, unlike those with diabetes, they usually have no symptoms at all. So in most cases, insulin resistance is not discovered until more serious health issues arise.

Insulin resistance, coupled with central obesity, high triglycerides, low levels of good cholesterol (HDL), and high blood pressure, is referred to as metabolic syndrome. This condition, sometimes called the "deadly quartet" by physicians, is a precursor to type 2 diabetes and cardiovascular disease, including heart attack and stroke. According to the National Health and Nutrition Examination Survey (NHANES), metabolic syndrome now affects a whopping 34 percent of Americans and is basically a time bomb ticking for those who have it.

AGEs Will Make You Age

Not only does excess sugar make you unhealthy and fat, it also causes you to age prematurely. The sugar that builds up in the blood and your body's tissues has nowhere to go, so it attaches to proteins, lipids, and nucleic acid in a process called glycation. These sugar complexes formed by glycation, known as advanced glycation end products (AGEs), are appropriately named, as they accelerate the aging process and contribute to age-related illnesses. AGEs accumulate, even in healthy people, but do so more quickly when blood sugars are high. AGEs cause cross-linking of such proteins as collagen and elastin that leave your muscles, tendons, and arteries stiff and your skin more wrinkled. AGEs have been found to be the culprit in age-related illnesses, including cardiovascular disease, kidney disease, Alzheimer's disease, and macular degeneration. AGEs have also been implicated in some of the most dreaded diabetic complications, including neuropathy, nephropathy, and cataracts. To put it bluntly, glycation is nothing short of a medical and beauty disaster. (We'll get into more detail on how sugar affects your skin in Chapter 4.)

Sugar as a Drug

If you're already following the 3-day Sugar Fix plan now, you'll know how dependent you are on the sweet stuff. And if the idea of living without sugar gives you the shakes, it makes total sense that you're addicted to sugar. Recent studies have shown interesting similarities between overconsumption of sugars and drug addiction. A study published in 2007 found that sugar cravings were even more demanding than cocaine cravings. And did you know that sugar can hold its own in the "drug" category? It's a substance that releases opioids (chemicals that produce euphoria) and dopamine (a neurotransmitter that helps control the brain's reward and pleasure centers). The release of the opioids and dopamine helps your body not feel pain at that moment and sends a pleasurable message to the brain—which is very similar to how the body responds to narcotics: Consuming sugar produces a happy feeling that makes you want to reach for it again and again. Sugar is so addictive, and we're eating such excess amounts of it, that scientists are recommending that sugar should be regulated by the government, the same way alcohol and tobacco are (and even large amounts of soda in New York City!).

Breaking the Habit

Take a minute to see how you are feeling on the 3-Day withdrawal. Do you feel as if you're really missing anything or are you actually starting to feel better already? With just a few days of sugar-free living behind you, your body and mind will start to feel better. Remember, this is a withdrawal and we're glad you're getting clean.

Now for Some Good News

By now, it must seem as if sugar is lurking in every dark corner, waiting to make a move. How do you know what's safe to eat? Relax! Because our ultimate goal is to avoid any spike in blood sugar, we've devised a system that takes into account foods' glycemic load, glycemic index, and the amount of fructose the food contains. These three key measures helped determine what foods to enjoy or what foods to avoid for this plan. We've gone a step further, too. Certain foods, herbs, and spices can actually help *reduce* the blood sugar spike that other foods may cause. That's more good news, because it means that you don't have to give up your favorite foods forever but instead can learn how to pair foods together to make them friendlier to your body and your skin. (We discuss this more in Chapter 7.)

Glycemic Index, Glycemic Load, and Fructose

Here's a quick tutorial on our three key measures.

Glycemic Index (GI). This is a numerical ranking system that measures how much your blood sugar rises after you eat a certain type of carbohydrate. A high GI number indicates that the carbohydrate was quickly broken down into glucose and will cause a blood sugar spike. Carbohydrates that break down slowly and have less of an effect on blood sugar have a low GI number. A low GI number is 55 or less, an intermediate number is 55 to 70 and a high GI is 70 or higher.

Glycemic Load (GL). This ranking system uses the glycemic index, plus takes into account portion size for the carbohydrates you're eating. This is important because if you eat a small amount of a high-GI food, you may affect your blood sugar more than if you were to eat a larger portion of food with a lower GI number. This is the best way to predict blood glucose values for a variety and differently sized portions of foods. A GL greater than 20 is considered high, 11 to 19 is a medium GL, and 10 or less is considered low. The foods on the Sugar Detox plan are all low or medium GI and GL. For more information on GI and GL, check out http://www.health.harvard.edu/newsweek/Glycemic_index_and_glycemic _load_for_100_foods.htm.

Fructose. Fructose is one of the three natural simple sugars found in fruits, vegetables, and honey. Its being a simple sugar means it is absorbed directly into the bloodstream during digestion. It is often used in processed foods in a form that mixes it with glucose to create high-fructose corn syrup (see page 35). Our Sugar Detox plan keeps your overall range of fructose under 20 grams a day (even from fruit).

By monitoring these three parameters, we have been able to create a diet plan that will have the lowest impact on your blood sugar levels. Keeping these levels stable and limiting the amount of unnecessary insulin production will prevent your body from storing extra fat and creating AGEs.

More on the F Word

How can something be considered bad if it comes from nature? That's a common question we get, regarding why we limit the amount of fructose you can have. Fructose is one of three major dietary monosaccharides (a monosaccharide is the simplest form of sugar), also known as single sugars. While, calorie for calorie, single sugars look the same to the body, fructose has been shown to have a different effect on the body's metabolism than do other single sugars. When the body is presented with fructose, it does not use it as an energy source. Instead, the fructose is metabolized exclusively by the liver, where some of it is turned into fat and stored. This is why consuming too much fructose from baked goods, sugary cereals, or products that contain high-fructose corn syrup contributes to development of a condition called nonalcoholic fatty liver disease (NAFLD). If fructose is consumed in liquid form, such as some fruit juices, sodas, or flavored milks, then the sugar reaches the liver even quicker and even more fat storage occurs.

Another thing that makes fructose different from glucose is that fructose does not cause the body to release insulin and causes the body to become resistant to the appetite-supressing hormone leptin. So it should come as no surprise that diets high in fructose cause excessive weight gain. Although fructose does not stimulate insulin secretion in the short term, long-term fructose consumption does cause a compensatory increase in insulin secretion. Diets high in fructose can cause insulin resistance, and ultimately, metabolic syndrome. A study published in the February 2012 edition of the *Journal of Nutrition* suggests that fructose consumption might increase cardiovascular risk factors simply because it increases visceral fat (remember, that's the bad internal fat). The study also showed that fructose consumption contributes to inflammation, cardiovascular diseases, and type 2 diabetes.

The final nail in the coffin for fructose is that it causes more AGEs than any other sugar does, making it a major player in glycation. Remember, AGEs accelerate the aging process, contribute to skin wrinkling, and cause certain age-related diseases.

Fructose—Let Us Count the Ways . . .

Not sure which foods are high in fructose? They include agave syrup, barbecue sauce, bread, breakfast cereals, brownies, cakes, caramel, commercial salad dressings, doughnuts, dried fruits, fruit juice, honey, ice cream and ices, jams and jellies, ketchup, pies, soft drinks, sports drinks, and tomato sauce.

While you may be thinking that fruit itself is a no-no, don't run away from the produce aisle just yet. Despite the considerable downside of fructose, certain fruits are allowed on the Sugar Detox plan. We don't allow it on the 3-Day Sugar Fix because it is a sugar, but we slowly start incorporating low-fructose, high-fiber fruit during Week 1 and increase your selection of fruits each week. We allow only low-fructose fruits in limited quantities for all four weeks, to help you get the best results possible. Some fruits, such as blueberries, are allowed starting in Week 2. They may be higher in fructose than we would like for this early week, but the potent antioxidants they contain are worth it. (More on that in Chapter 5.)

Avoid These Sugar Substitutes

Artificial Sweeteners

You might be thinking that if sugar is a big no-no here, then why not use artificial sweeteners? Well, don't reach for the pink, blue, or yellow packet yet. As it turns out, you can't fool Mother Nature. Plenty of research has shown the negative side effects linked to artificial sweeteners. Research hot off the presses, for example, reveals that artificial sweeteners have almost the exact same effects on the body as the real stuff does: When sugar receptors (found in the mouth, gut, and pancreas) get tripped, they signal the brain to get ready for a sugar blast. The body reacts in turn by absorbing more real sugar, triggering insulin production and turning sugar into fat. And guess what? These super sweet little chemicals stimulate the same receptors that real sugar does, and with the same results. To make it even worse, artificial sweeteners

---

Sugar by Any Other Name . . .

We know now that sugar comes in many different forms, but sugar is sneaky. Don't be fooled by labels that say "no sugar added" or "contains only natural sugars"; they are all just different disguises worn by sugar. Always read the ingredient list and check to see whether any of the following words are listed. If yes, then the product contains sugar: agave syrup, brown rice syrup, brown sugar, cane sugar, caramel, corn sweetener, corn syrup, corn syrup solids, date sugar, dextrose, fructose, fruit juice concentrate, glucose, high-fructose corn syrup, honey, invert sugar, lactose, maltose, malt, malt syrup, maple sugar, maple syrup, molasses, raw sugar, rice syrup, sorghum syrup, sucrose, sweetened carob powder, turbinado.

---

increase your appetite in general, so you consume even more calories. So as you can see, these imposters actually cause you to absorb more sugars, store fat, and gain weight. Is it any surprise that they are now considered just as dangerous as the real stuff?

Other dangers of artificial sweeteners include possible links to cancer, headaches, seizures, weight gain, memory loss, bloating, anxiety, skin rashes, and so much more. One of the more recent artificial sweeteners happens to be a completely man-made substance manufactured by a company best known for its baby body wash and swabs to clean ears: Splenda was created with the use of chlorine and some extra chemistry. A study showed that this chlorinated sweetener alters the gut microflora that are prudent to healthy living. Very few studies have been done on the long-term safety of Splenda or any other artificial sweetener to date, so we think it's best to avoid them at all costs.

Agave

Agave nectar used to be the go-to sweetener for people watching their blood sugar levels because it has a very low glycemic index. The problem with agave is that it is composed mainly of fructose. In fact, agave, although given the health halo because it's natural and from a plant, has more fructose than docs any other common sweetener—even more than high-fructose corn syrup!

High Fructose Corn Syrup

Plenty of controversy surrounds high-fructose corn syrup (HFCS), a calorie-providing sweetener used in everything from soft drinks to condiments to packaged foods. Food manufacturers often include this sugary ingredient as not only an affordable sweetener but as a preservative, to help foods maintain a longer shelf life. While research as yet has not shown significant differences between the metabolism of HFCS and sugar (sucrose), the problem is that HFCS is mainly found in foods with little to no nutritional value and empty calories. Therefore, HFCS is not part of any healthy diet, especially the Sugar Detox.

A Spoonful of Sugar . . .

There are many reasons to always read ingredient labels because it's amazing what has sugar hiding in plain sight. Common pharmacy products that often contain sugar include cough drops and throat lozenges, vitamin supplements, and many over-the-counter medications, such as cough syrups. Even prescription medications in pill or liquid form may contain sweeteners, such as lactose.

Now you know why sugar is the bad guy and how our plan is mapped out for you. Later in the book, you'll learn why we're having you eat what you're eating and how food can be the best medicine! But next, let's talk about skin.

SWEET SUCCESS
Jonathan

Jonathan's primary-care physician referred him to B Nutritious because his blood sugar levels were high and his doctor was ready to put him on blood sugar medication. Jonathan was already on high doses of statin medication to lower his cholesterol, when he came into Brooke's office. A lawyer, Jonathan wanted things to happen quickly through diet or he would just go on the medication. "It's easier and quicker," he said. Brooke realized that Jonathon was a big snacker—he was constantly eating chips, pretzels, and even 100-calorie packs (which he would eat at least three at a time). By increasing the amount of protein and fiber through his day, while reducing his sugar intake through the Sugar Detox plan, Jonathan was surprised how quickly and effectively the diet changed his habits and his health. "I was fine taking medication before, but now I realize I can control not only my blood sugar but also my cholesterol with the Sugar Detox."

4

Sugar: Not So Sweet
for Your Skin, Either

Are you staring in the mirror these days, seeing your mother looking back at you? If so, you're not alone. The science behind aging has shown that a good bit of what happens or doesn't happen to us as we grow old is a result of our genetics. Dermatologists call this natural, or intrinsic, aging; and it is the reason that people can say, if you want to know what a woman is going to look like as she ages, just look at her mother. But it's the other type of aging that we are concerned with, an aging that can be prevented. Called extrinsic aging, this type of aging occurs mostly because of our own bad behaviors.

Everyone knows that excessive sun exposure accelerates the aging process. The ultraviolet A rays (UVAs) you get from indoor tanning are the absolute worst when it comes to skin aging because these long-wavelength beams penetrate deep into the dermis, damaging the supporting structure of the skin and causing wrinkling. Interesting new data has shown that pollution takes a toll on your skin as well. Women living in cities where they are exposed to high levels of pollution have more wrinkles and blotchy pigmentation than do those living in more rural settings—yet another reason to leave the rat race of the big city and enjoy some time in the country! And let's not forget to mention that those cigarettes that you may still smoke will send skin aging into overdrive (yep, even one or two regular cigarettes will show up on your face). In short, all of these environmental insults to the skin contribute to extrinsic aging.

Food and Your Face

Food is the most recent addition to the list of things that contribute to extrinsic aging. Nutricosmetics is the study of how nutrition and your diet affects your appearance and is a subject of growing interest among dermatologists. Early researchers in this field reasoned that if we can reduce the chances of heart disease, diabetes, high blood pressure, and other age-related illnesses by dietary interventions, then surely we can improve the way people look as well. Studies have now confirmed that they were right. Dermatologists now appreciate that nutrition is an important factor in extrinsic aging, and as the word gets out, using dietary interventions to improve appearance is gaining momentum. For example, a recent study showed that eating colorful fruits and vegetables, which are full of antioxidants, can improve skin health and appearance.

Our scientifically developed diet and skin regimen is designed to protect and repair your skin from the ravages of extrinsic aging.

The Telltale Signs of Skin Aging

What's interesting is that a dermatologist, just by looking at your skin, can actually tell the difference between the aging that occurs as a result of the passage of time and that which is the result of environmental factors. Naturally aged skin looks totally different from extrinsically aged skin. Naturally aged skin has no discolorations at all, is thin and finely wrinkled, and looks kind of like tissue paper. This is a stark contrast to extrinsic aging that leaves your skin looking a lot like those leathery babes you see in Miami Beach. In extrinsic aging, the skin is discolored with large brown spots and freckles, has deep, coarse wrinkles, and appears sallow. Another striking feature of extrinsic aging is unsightly sagging, because sun exposure and poor nutrition cause skin to lose elasticity.

Why does extrinsically aged skin look so bad? Well, the problem here is that subjecting your skin to a combination of sun exposure, pollution, and poor nutrition leaves it virtually defenseless. Furthermore, the repair mechanisms that your skin relies on become disabled by the onslaught, so that the damage cannot be repaired. This is why the prevention of extrinsic aging is so important.

The Anatomy of a Wrinkle

To understand what causes wrinkles, you have to know the anatomy of the skin. Skin is comprised of two layers: the upper layer (the epidermis) and the lower layer (the dermis). The supporting structure of the skin, located in the dermis, is composed of collagen and elastin fibers. These are proteins that are embedded in a soft substance called hyaluronic acid. Hyaluronic acid is what makes your skin plump, while collagen and elastin are what help keep the skin firm and tight.

After environmental exposure (think sun here), the elastin fibers become frayed and fragmented. This process, called solar elastosis, is unique to sun exposure. Solar elastosis not only causes the skin to lose elasticity; it also gives the skin a yellowish cast. Recent studies have determined that this yellow cast can be attributed to AGEs that are present in sun-damaged skin.

Environmental exposure likewise causes collagen fibers to deteriorate and diminish. Where does the collagen go? Does it just vanish into thin air or does it disappear slowly? The answer is actually a little bit of both. There is always some collagen being formed while older collagen is being broken down, a process called collagen homeostasis. However, when skin ages, and especially when it is subjected to environmental exposure and poor nutrition, the scales begin to tip, with more collagen breaking down than forming. This leaves the supporting structure of the skin weak, which leads to wrinkling and sagging. This is also why wounds heal with more slowly as we age. An essential step in healing any injury to the skin is the formation of new collagen.

Free Radicals Gone Wild

The delicate balance of collagen homeostasis is profoundly affected by free radicals. Free radicals, also found in naturally aged skin, are produced in much larger quantities in extrinsically aged skin. Sun exposure, pollution, cigarettes, and eating the wrong foods can cause free radicals to form.

Free radicals are derived from oxygen molecules that have lost an electron. Free radicals are greedy: When they lose an electron, they try to repair themselves by stealing one from another molecule. In effect, they become whole again while leaving another molecule short of an electron, creating a vicious cycle. Free radicals act like a Ping-Pong ball run amok, bouncing around inside cells and tissues while damaging everything in their path, including cell membranes, proteins such as collagen and elastin, and even DNA.

Free radicals also turn on and off certain cellular processes within cells. In terms of skin, they break down collagen and weaken the supporting structure of the dermis. Free radicals also lead to the production in the skin of a number of inflammatory mediators, molecules that turn on inflammation that results in further breakdown of collagen and elastin fibers, which ultimately accelerates aging.

Antioxidants to the Rescue

Luckily, young healthy skin has a sophisticated protective mechanism. Antioxidants can neutralize free radicals in the skin and elsewhere in the body. Naturally occurring antioxidants in the skin include vitamin C, vitamin E, coenzyme Q10, glutathione, and alpha-lipoic acid (ALA). There is also a group of enzymes that function as antioxidants, including superoxide dismutase (SOD), glutathione peroxidase (GPX1), and catalase (CAT). You may actually recognize some of these antioxidant terms, as many of them are found in anti-aging skin-care products—the rationale being that applying antioxidants directly to the skin in an absorbent cream will protect it from free radicals.

Prevention becomes even more important as skin ages, because antioxidants that occur naturally become less plentiful and free radicals more numerous resulting in what is called oxidative stress. The foods you eat on the Sugar Detox plan, along with our daily dermal detox regimen (see Chapter 9), will help you reduce free radical formation while boosting your antioxidant defense system.

What's Sugar Got to Do with It?

Most of what we know about sugar and skin aging comes from the study of diabetics. In the late 1970s, researchers began to look at diabetics in an attempt to explain why they suffered such grave medical problems. The scientists knew that diabetics were more prone to develop such conditions as heart disease, kidney failure, eye problems, and nerve damage, and that they also experienced poor wound healing. Some diabetics even develop an unusual type of skin condition that leaves the skin stiff. So physicians began to ask themselves, what is the common thread among all these diabetic complications?

What they discovered was that almost all of the complications diabetics suffered from could be explained by glycation. As we mentioned earlier, glycation is a chemical process that occurs when blood sugar levels are high and circulating sugars bind to proteins, lipids, and nucleic acids, forming compounds called AGEs. AGEs are found in the kidneys, brain, nervous tissue, and—no surprise—the skin. Researchers also discovered that some of the most damaging AGEs found in diabetics are glycated collagen and elastin. When these soft, supple fibers are glycated, they become excessively cross-linked and stiff. It is believed that glycated collagen and elastin are responsible for hardening of the arteries, poor wound healing, and perhaps even the skin stiffness seen in diabetics. This explains why diabetics who control their blood sugar carefully—and thus have fewer AGEs—suffer far fewer long-term complications than do those who allow their blood sugar to fluctuate.

AGEs and Your Skin

It's important to understand that AGEs are not only found in the skin of diabetics but in everyone's, as a result of both natural and extrinsic aging. Glycation starts when you are in your mid-thirties and rapidly increases with age. Here's the thing: How fast you accumulate glycated collagen and elastin is directly related to your dietary intake of sugar. In other words, the more sugar and refined carbohydrates you consume, the more glycated collagen and elastin you will have and the older your skin will appear. Sun exposure also increases the rate at which collagen and elastin are glycated because oxidative stress puts glycation into overdrive. Glycated collagen is stiff and rigid and sugar-coated elastin loses its snap leaving skin sagging and wrinkled. And because it is very difficult to remove or repair glycated collagen and elastin once it has formed, the earlier you start your prevention program, the better off you will be (if you're getting started a little later, not to worry—our diet and dermal detox will have you looking years younger, no matter when you begin it).

Beware of Browning

It is important to understand that AGEs have two dietary sources. Some AGEs are formed as a result of your sugar intake; others are the result of certain cooking techniques, such as frying, grilling, and roasting. That golden brown skin of a Thanksgiving turkey or the yummy brown crust on bread is the result of glycation. (In cooking, this glycation is called the Maillard reaction, which occurs when foods are heated at a high temperature in the absence of water, causing the production of AGEs. Boiling, poaching, and steaming do not produce AGEs because water-based cooking does not involve browning.) These latter AGEs further glycate collagen and other proteins and ramp up inflammation and oxidative stress. In other words, the AGEs caused by improper cooking are just as damaging as those formed by sugars, and maybe even more. Dietary AGEs also alter the bacteria that live in your gut, interfering with the absorption of important vitamins and nutrients. This compounds the problem, as many of these vitamins and nutrients need to be used in the body to inhibit AGE formation. The bottom line: Just as you know how bad it is for your skin to bake in the sun, don't brown your foods!

Putting It All Together

So, do people who eat too much sugar really look older? The answer is a resounding YES! In a large study published in the journal *AGE*, 602 people were examined by independent evaluators. Healthy people with lower blood sugars typically looked a year younger than did those with higher blood sugars, and a year and a half younger than did diabetics of the same age. The authors of this study suggest that looking better might give people a motivation to follow a nutritious and healthy diet that is low in added sugars. (We agree and our program is designed to do just that.)

Too much sugar also has another negative effect on skin: Simply put, it makes skin unhealthy. Skin is our largest organ; one of its main functions, called barrier function, is to protect us from environmental insults such as pollution, dirt, bacteria, and fungi. Anything that disrupts the epidermal barrier leaves us more vulnerable to skin irritation and infections. Some very interesting recent studies have shown that long-term hyperglycemia (too much sugar in the blood) leaves skin more vulnerable. This explains why diabetics and others with long-standing hyperglycemia so often suffer with dry skin. This is why controlling your blood sugar is so important if you want healthy skin.

Sugar and the Breakout Blues

Acne affects an estimated 40 to 50 million people in the United States every year. This incidence of acne peaks in adolescence, when it affects a whopping 85 percent of teens. Fifteen to 20 percent of teen sufferers will go on to have acne as adults. Dermatologists are seeing more adult acne patients now than ever—and far more adult women experience acne than do men. Teens and adults with acne will do almost anything to clear their skin, spending over 2 billion dollars every year on over-the-counter medications. They also frequent dermatologist offices, asking for prescription medications and such procedures as chemical peels, lasers, or light treatments, in hopes of finding a cure.

SWEET SUCCESS
Deborah

Deborah came to see Dr. Farris five months before her daughter's wedding. "I just want to do anything short of cosmetic surgery that will make me look better." She admitted to having gained 20 or so pounds since she had gone through menopause. "I can't seem to lose a pound." Further questioning revealed that she had quit exercising due to her busy work schedule and she admitted her diet wasn't what she called "the healthiest"—she ate "a lot on the road in coffee shops and other small, quick, pickup-type restaurants." Dr. Farris noted that she had significant skin aging, sagging along the jaw line and neck, spots and dark discolorations on the cheeks, some forehead and eyelid laxity, and dark circles under her eyes. She began to review Deborah's diet with her. A typical breakfast was coffee with artificial sweetener and a bagel; lunch, either a wrap with chicken or turkey; and was primarily meat and potatoes at dinner. Deborah admitted to being a "carboholic" and acknowledged breads as her guilty pleasure. "I like sweets but only have dessert when I'm out to dinner."

Dr. Farris outlined a treatment plan for Deborah that included the 3-Day Sugar Fix and the four-week program. She prescribed an antioxidant serum to be used daily to protect her skin and control skin glycation, and a series of chemical peels to improve uneven pigmentation and skin radiance. In just two weeks, Deborah had lost 5 pounds and was feeling more energetic. She also noted that her skin was brighter and that the patchy dryness she had suffered with for years was gone. Dr. Farris performed biweekly chemical peels and instructed Deborah on selecting a proper repairing moisturizer for her skin type. At the end of the four-week program, Deborah had lost 8 pounds and reported that her skin never looked better. Encouraged by her success, Deborah now controls her sugar intake as part of a comprehensive program to fight skin aging.

What causes acne? Stress is known to contribute to breakouts, but the answer is more complicated than we originally thought. Dermatologists have always known that hormonal fluctuations that occur

Lynn, a forty-two-year-old account executive, had never experienced acne during her teen years. Over the past several years, though, she began to have what she described as underground pimples that seemed to last forever. She admitted to having a lot of stress at work and to having flare-ups of acne that seemed to be related to her menstrual cycle. "The week before my period, the acne gets so bad on my chin that I can't even cover it." She had tried over-the-counter products containing benzoyl peroxide and a salicylic acid, which didn't seem to help all that much. Dr. Farris discussed the causes of adult acne with Lynn and suggested that she keep a food diary of what she was eating for one month. Much to her surprise, Lynn realized that her sweet tooth got the best of her during the latter part of her cycle. In other words, at that time of the month, she was eating way more candy and sweet stuff than she realized. Dr. Farris started Lynn on the Sugar Detox right away. She also prescribed a topical antibiotic and an oil-control lotion, and recommended yoga to help with stress. At her four-week follow-up visit, Lynn had lost 8 pounds and was feeling more confident about her skin. By using a holistic approach to Lynn's problem, Dr. Farris not only cleared her skin but also helped her manage her stress and lose weight.

throughout life are a major factor contributing to the development of acne. Our oil glands are under hormonal influence; it is androgen, or male hormones that turn on oil production. Androgens are present in both male and females during puberty and are the reason kids of this age are troubled with oily skin, oily hair, and acne. Genetics also play a major role, especially in patients who experience more severe types of acne, such as cystic acne. In other words, if your parents or siblings had cystic acne, you are far more likely to develop it.

The relationship between diet and acne has been the subject of great controversy among dermatologists for years. In the early 1950s,

Acne Can Be More Than Just a Blemish

Acne can be the sign of more serious hormonal issues, including poly-cystic ovarian syndrome (PCOS), which affects an estimated 15 per-cent of all women during their reproductive years (PCOS produces irregular menstrual cycles and is a major cause of infertility if left un-treated). This is a genetically determined hormonal disorder—most women diagnosed with PCOS have a close relative with this condition. Studies have shown that women with PCOS have higher levels of in-sulin (after a sugar load) than most due to insulin resistance. The ovaries produce excessive amounts of androgens, which in turn can produce acne and grow facial hair. Women with PCOS are also prone to weight gain, which is due to the fat-storing caused by excess in-sulin; they are additionally at risk for heart disease, atherosclerosis, and metabolic syndrome. Early intervention and proper treatment is essential to prevent these problems. While there is no cure for PCOS, it can be effectively treated with a comprehensive treatment plan that includes medications and a diet such as the Sugar Detox that limits processed food, added sugars, and refined carbohydrates, all of which will effectively lower blood sugar.

textbooks of dermatology contained information suggesting that patients with acne avoid chocolate, fats, sweets, and soft drinks. These dietary recommendations were removed from the textbooks when studies failed to show a definitive relationship between these foods and breakouts. Recently, however, dermatologists have finally put together the pieces of the puzzle—and sugar has been fingered as one of the chief culprits, after all. It started with a simple observation that in non-Westernized island cultures, where people basically eat what they hunt and harvest, acne is virtually nonexistent, even in kids who are going through pu-berty. In these societies, the diet consists primarily of fresh vegetables, fruits, and proteins, and there are no processed foods or added sugars. How these more natural diets were protecting teens from acne remained

SWEET SUCCESS
Kathy

Kathy is a fashion executive who struggled with her weight for years. Her menstrual cycles had always been somewhat irregular and she often went three to four months between periods. She saw her gynecologist, who ran blood work that confirmed the diagnosis of PCOS. Kathy decided to see a dermatologist for some recommendations on routine skin care and acne treatment. Dr. Farris reviewed Kathy's medical history, including her blood work. Dr. Farris explained that by controlling sugar, Kathy could improve her weight and her acne. Kathy started the Sugar Detox 31-day program. Much to Kathy's surprise, she lost 5 pounds in two weeks. "This is the first time I have been able to lose any weight in forever." Today, Kathy remains committed to staying on a low-sugar diet. She now realizes that with her hormonal condition, following a diet low in added sugars and refined carbohydrates is an important part of the long-term strategy for treating her problem.

a mystery until several years ago, when research demonstrated that high-sugar diets and high insulin levels trigger a hormonal cascade that causes acne. These hormones stimulate oil production and increase proliferation of skin cells that can block pores.

This explains why cutting-edge dermatologists now treat acne with both medications and a low-glycemic-index diet. We have already seen the benefits of a reduced-sugar diet; in addition, the Sugar Detox helps turn off the hormonal storm that can cause acne . . . which is why so many of our patients with acne get better on our plan.

5

What to Eat

"The Sugar Detox changed my entire view on what I eat and how I look at food. After completing the 31-day plan I realized I had been constantly snacking on sugary foods that were not only unhealthy but would be just a temporary fix for my hunger. After starting Sugar Detox I found myself with more energy, fewer cravings, and an overall better attitude about both my mind and body. I had no idea I was making such poor choices in my diet and in my snacks, but after following Sugar Detox for just a few weeks, I was able to shop at any food store or order in any restaurant and choose foods that fit within the diet and continued to make me lose weight and feel better about myself. The Sugar Detox is so easy to follow and gives such amazing results, you are able to stick with it past the thirty-one days."

What was important to us as we created this diet plan for you, was to be as clear as possible about what you should be eating. We wanted to focus on the foods you *can* eat, rather than making it feel like deprivation by telling you all the things you *can't* have. We also knew it would be helpful for you to understand *why* we suggest eating certain foods and avoiding others. Our goal was to group the foods into a few simple categories, to make it easier for you to make a choice of when you need to eat a protein, a fat, a starch, or even a dessert. (You'll see that some groups overlap; for instance, a nut is both a fat and a protein, so it can be used for your fat for the day or as a vegetarian protein option.) We also highlight some specific foods—our all-stars—that have superior health benefits.

If you are concerned about food preparation, rest assured that this diet does not require preparing every meal entirely from scratch (see pages 233–239 for approved brands of packaged foods). And in addition to providing more than fifty recipes (see Chapter 13), we encourage you to dine out without fear (see Chapter 12). A basic understanding of the food groups will ground you in your many meal options.

Vegetables

You'll notice that the Sugar Detox, regardless of whether you're doing the 3-Day Sugar Fix or any of the four weeks, is pretty veggie heavy. In fact, you can eat an unlimited amount of veggies while on this plan, as long as they're on the approved list. The great thing about these Sugar Detox–approved vegetables is that they have virtually no impact on your blood sugar levels, while providing you with lots of essential vitamins, minerals, antioxidants, and fiber. So, when in doubt, veg out!

While our list of approved vegetables is relatively long, it's nowhere near complete, compared to all the amazing veggie options that do exist. We kept it short to make things a little easier for you—no one wants to walk through the supermarket with a shopping list that's three pages long. But if any of your favorite veggies weren't included, you can most certainly add them—just make sure they're not on the no-no's list (see page 75).

Green Leafy Vegetables

We might sound like your mother constantly telling you to eat your veggies, but she was on to something. Green leafy vegetables, such as spinach and dark-colored lettuce, are nutrition powerhouses and a staple of the Sugar Detox. These green beauties contain essential vitamins, minerals, phytochemicals, antioxidants, and fiber. Leafy greens not only have little to no sugar, but have a healthy effect on blood sugar levels because the fiber in the greens actually slows down digestion, preventing any sugar spikes. A study published in the *British Medical Journal* also showed that eating more green leafy vegetables could significantly lower the risk of developing Type 2 diabetes. If you are following our plan correctly, you will certainly be meeting your green leafy vegetable daily quota!

> *Sweet Talk*
> BA says:
>
> *"Is your body slow to adjust to all the veggies? Eat your salads well chopped—it makes them a little more gentle on the belly!"*

If you weren't a big veggie eater prior to starting the Sugar Detox, you may find that your belly needs to go through an adjustment period. All this fiber, while so healthy for you, does make an impact on your gastrointestinal track, so start slowly with cooked vegetables, versus raw, to aid with this transition. Have some peppermint tea with meals to prevent any unpleasant bloating or too many runs to the bathroom from this unaccustomed roughage.

Cruciferous Vegetables

Other green veggies, such as broccoli, cabbage, kale, and bok choy, as well as cauliflower, are all part of the cruciferous vegetable family. These amazing veggies deliver a one-two punch, as they are packed with cancer-fighting properties and have minimal sugar and calories. A review of research by the *Journal of the American Dietetic Association* (its parent organization is now known as the Academy of Nutrition and Dietetics) back in the '90s found that 70 percent or more of the studies found a link between cruciferous vegetables and protection against cancer. As if that wasn't enough to eat them, the beta-carotene in many of these vegetables contributes to the growth and repair of the body's tissues and can protect your skin from sun damage, which can lead to premature aging.

Sea Vegetables

Sea vegetables, commonly known as seaweed, aren't just for sushi rolls anymore. Neither plants nor animals but in the same family as algae, sea vegetables come in thousands of different varieties and are often categorized by color. They contain tons of nutrients, including iodine, a hard-to-get mineral that is considered so important to life functioning that many countries, including the United States, add it to table salt. Sea vegetables also contain significant amounts of iron (great for vegetarians), magnesium, calcium, B vitamins, and even vitamin C. They're low in calories, high in fiber, and have basically no impact on your blood sugar. Sea vegetables can be found in health food stores, specialty markets, and ethnic grocers, as well as the Asian foods aisle in larger supermarkets. Common varieties are kelp (also known as kombu), wakame, and nori. Kelp can be used as a noodle substitute, and is great in soups and stir-fries. Wakame is tasty in miso soup or roasted and sprinkled on salads. And nori, the seaweed typically found in sushi rolls, can be eaten on its own as a crunchy snack. These undersea delights score a big punch for flavor and nutritional value.

Sweet Talk

BA says:

"Don't get fooled by seaweed salads at Japanese restaurants— they're loaded with sugar!"

Proteins

This isn't a diet plan where you gnaw on huge pieces of meat like a caveman, although you do get to eat a significant amount of protein. Whether your protein sources are lean meats, seafood, nuts, or legumes, protein is an essential part of the Sugar Detox. It keeps you full, helps you feel satisfied, and most important here, keeps your blood sugar stable. Note that the Sugar Detox can be followed by both vegetarians and vegans; see the box on page 4 for more info about vegetarian and vegan-friendly substitutions.

Lean Meats, Poultry and Pork

Because lean red meat, poultry, and pork don't contain any sugar on their own (unless you use a sweetened marinade), they are safe foods for the Sugar Detox.

RED MEAT

Red meat shouldn't be eaten more than twice a week and ideally should come from grass-fed animals. Grass-fed beef has been shown to have a higher percentage of protein over saturated fat, compared to corn-fed beef. While even grass-fed beef does contain some saturated fats, it also contains conjugated linoleic acid (CLA) and is a healthy source of the mineral chromium. CLA, a type of fatty acid, has been shown in numerous studies to have a positive effect on weight management, mainly by reducing total body fat and increasing lean body mass. Chromium, an essential mineral that we must get from either our food or a supplement, helps insulin function properly, as well as aids the body in metabolizing carbohydrates, and therefore sugar, more effectively. Bison is a great red meat option from which you still get your chromium but without as much fat as from a regular piece of red meat.

POULTRY AND PORK

Chicken, turkey, or pork are a great source of protein and contain little fat, so they are a staple of the Sugar Detox. The protein in these meats keeps you full and helps slow down the absorption of whatever sugar or starch is eaten with it, making it a great pairing to anything that could spike your blood sugar (see more in Chapter 7). Just make sure you're opting for healthy, natural protein sources, eating sparingly of others, such as bacon, ham, sausages, hot dogs, and cold cuts.

Fish and Shellfish

Seafood is a great protein option, as it has little to no effect on your blood sugar when you eat it. Even better, certain fish such as salmon contain essential fatty acids (which are fatty acids that are necessary for human health, but the body can't produce them) that have an amazing impact on heart health. In fact, an extremely large study called the Physicians' Health Study found that men with the highest blood levels of these essential fatty acids had an 80 percent lower risk of dying from a cardiovascular-related disease or event than those who had lower levels. Essential fatty acids, especially DHA (which is derived from omega-3), can also help prevent insulin resistance by improving cell sensitivity to insulin. They are also the building blocks for the natural moisturizers in your skin and help keep skin hydrated. (Omega-3s are also available from nonseafood sources. For more on this, see page 56.)

Fish and shellfish are staples of a Mediterranean diet. This way of eating has long been touted for its cardiovascular benefits and protection, but it's also been shown to have a great impact on blood sugar. A study published in the *New England Journal of Medicine* compared results of three diets: a low-fat plan with restricted calories, a Mediterranean diet with restricted calories, and a low-carbohydrate plan without caloric restriction. The only diet that showed a positive effect on blood glucose was the Mediterranean diet. The protein and healthy fats found in fish are good for fighting inflammation and keeping skin hydrated.

Legumes and Nuts

Legumes and nuts have amazing health benefits. They are a great vegetarian source of protein, contain plenty of fiber, and are often inexpensive and easy to prepare.

LEGUMES

Legumes (peas; beans, including soybeans; lentils; and peanuts) do contain some carbohydrates, but because of their makeup, and more important, their fiber content, they can help manage or lower blood sugar levels.

Lentils especially are packed with both soluble and insoluble dietary fiber: The soluble fiber helps to slow down the absorption of sugar molecules that lentils contain; the insoluble fiber is passed through the digestive tract without actually being "seen" by the body as a carbohydrate or sugar. The fiber in lentils and other legumes slows down the entire digestive process in a positive way, so you stay fuller longer and more satisfied while keeping your blood sugar stable.

Soybeans are a great vegetarian protein option. They can be eaten plain as edamame, or as tofu or tempeh. Soybeans should be eaten only in these forms, as soy can also be highly processed. Processed soy can be found everywhere, often in the form of soy protein isolate—textured vegetable protein (TVP)—and should be avoided. It is best to eat soybeans and soy products organically whenever possible.

NUTS

Nuts, such as almonds, cashews, pistachios, walnuts, pecans, and macadamias, are a great snack. They're super portable, have a long shelf life, and can also help on those days you have the munchies. Their protein, unsaturated healthy fat (see also page 56), and fiber make nuts an amazing powerhouse in a small package. Nuts are especially rich in an amino acid called L-arginine, which might help improve cardiovascular health. Adding nuts to your meals is a great way of food combining (more about this in Chapter 7) so that the entire meal is digested slower and you have less sugar spikes. Nuts are also a great source of magnesium, calcium, and potassium, while low in sodium (provided they are unsalted). A high intake of these minerals together can protect against bone breakdown, hypertension, insulin resistance, and cardiovascular disease. Magnesium is essential for overall good health and is absolutely required from the diet to help maintain constant levels in the body. While magnesium is needed

> *Sweet **Talk***
> **BA says:**
>
> *"Nut servings vary depending on the nut—23 almonds, 21 hazelnuts, 18 cashews, 19 pecans, 14 walnuts, 11 macadamias, and 49 pistachios."*

for over three hundred different kinds of biochemical reactions in the body, it also helps regulate blood sugar levels and is considered an all-star nutrient for the Sugar Detox.

Fats

It may seem counterintuitive to eat fats when you're following a diet, but healthy fats are an essential part of the Sugar Detox. The Mediterranean diet is renowned for its healthy fats, primarily from nuts, seeds, and olives, which are essential in your diet. Monounsaturated fatty acids (MUFAs) and polyunsaturated fatty acids (PUFAs), which also include those omega-3 fatty acids that we discussed previously as pertaining to fish and shellfish, have been shown to help lower blood cholesterol levels, have cardiovascular protective benefits, and can benefit blood sugar control. In a study published in 2005, a diet high in healthy fats was shown to help with insulin resistance, probably because fat can't be broken down into glucose. Although it might sound counterintuitive, a diet rich in monounsaturated fats may also prevent the accumulation of abdominal fat, a major indicator of insulin resistance/metabolic syndrome. In addition, fat can actually curb your appetite, by triggering the release of a hormone called cholecystokinin, which causes the feeling of fullness. Choosing the right kind of fats to include in your diet is a major component of the Sugar Detox and that's why there is always a minimum requirement of three servings a day, right from the start.

Seeds

Seeds are often underestimated for their amazing nutrition power that's packed into each tiny little nugget. Flaxseeds are well known for their healthy impact on cardiovascular health and their ability to lower cholesterol; there is also new evidence that flaxseeds can improve blood sugar levels. Chia seeds, flax's lesser-known cousin, are even more talented. Similar to poppy seeds in appearance, chia is high in protein, loaded with fiber, and full of omega-3 fatty acids—these latter two components are what make chia effective in actually lowering blood sugar. There is even some evidence that chia seeds can help reduce belly fat, the type that contributes to insulin resistance. Other seeds, such as sunflower seeds, hemp seeds, and pumpkin seeds, contain a type of healthy fat called linoleic acid. A study published in the *American Journal of Clinical Nutrition* linked this fatty acid to supporting weight loss, especially in the abdominal area, and to lowering glucose levels in postmenopausal women.

Nuts

We discussed nuts as a protein, but they are fats, too. Almost every kind of nut contains protein, fiber, and healthy fats but no sugar, which makes them a great snack or meal addition. Eating nuts can lower your risk for cardiovascular disease, because their fat component interferes with cholesterol absorption, which helps reduce the LDL levels in the bloodstream. Pairing nuts with other healthy fats, fiber, and protein can help slow down the absorption of sugar (especially in meals that may not be a Sugar Detox–approved option and so, full of sugar)— think of it as a buddy system. (See Chapter 7 for more discussion of food combining.)

PISTACHIO NUTS

A study published in the *European Journal of Clinical Nutrition* found that consuming about 2 ounces of pistachios along with high-carbohydrate foods significantly lowered postmeal blood glucose response. Pistachios have been shown specifically to help prevent spikes in blood sugar when eaten with a higher-sugar meal.

The pistachio study proposed that nuts, which are low in sugars and carbohydrates while containing protein and fat, may replace the sugar and carbohydrate content of some meals, for a positive impact on blood sugar reactions. Pistachios also contain a special type of vitamin E called gamma-tocopherol, which is thought to be a cancer fighter.

Fruits That Contain Fat

Not many fruits contain fat, but two of our all-star foods do: avocados and coconuts. These fatty fruits have gotten bad raps in the past and we're here to set the record straight!

AVOCADO

This fatty fruit is truly an all-star! It contains twenty essential nutrients, including a nice dose of fiber and healthy fats, all while having a low glycemic-index rating and containing barely any fructose or starch at all. The monounsaturated fat in avocados has heart-healthy benefits and anti-inflammatory properties. Avocados are a great source of magnesium, a mineral (also found in nuts, leafy greens, and fish) that has been linked to a 10 to 20 percent decrease in the risk of developing diabetes in women. Avocados are also rich in sterols, compounds that have been shown to lower cholesterol. We love avocados in smoothies for a healthy fat boost, added to salads for a creamy texture and fat satiating, and on their own as a snack with a squeeze of lemon juice.

COCONUT

This poor fruit was vilified during the fat-free diet craze in the '90s and is still working to prove it's not the bad guy here. Because the fat in coconuts is a saturated fat, it's gotten grouped together with fatty cuts of meat, butter, and ice cream. However, not all saturated fats are created equal. Coconut meat is low in sugar, has a low glycemic index and load, and contains a type of fat that's healthy for you and can be used for energy! Coconut meat and coconut oil contain a type of fat called lauric acid, which has been touted for its healing benefits because the body converts it to monolaurin, which has antiviral and antibacterial properties.

The main star of coconut oil is its medium-chain fatty acids (MCFAs). The difference between coconut oil and other oils is the size of their fat molecules. Common vegetable oils and the majority of the fats you consume contain large molecules of fat called large-chain fatty acids (LCFAs). Because of LCFAs' size, it's too difficult for your body to break them down and so they generally get stored as fat. MCFAs, however, are small, easily digested, and used as energy in the body. A number of studies have found that the MCFAs in coconut oil can't be easily converted into stored fats, nor can the body use them to make larger fat molecules. Another study showed that dietetic supplementation with coconut oil does not cause weight gain and, in fact, promotes a reduction in abdominal obesity. Even more proof was published in the international journal *Diabetes* in 2009 that showed that a diet rich in coconut oil could protect against insulin resistance and help prevent the accumulation of body fat.

Coconut oil is perfect to cook with, as it's very heat stable. Often when you're cooking with oils, a high temperature turns them into trans-fatty acids or they start smoking too quickly, which turns them rancid or into unhealthy free radicals. Coconut oil is perfect for sautéing veggies or scrambling eggs, or in a stir-fry.

A note about coconut water: This beverage is not the same as coconut milk or oil, which are derived from coconut flesh. Coconut water—the liquid that forms naturally in the center of a whole coconut—helps with hydration and keeping your electrolytes balanced. Pure coconut water is a great, low-sugar way to rehydrate after a very sweaty exercise session. However, note that coconut waters that contain added flavorings or juices are not Sugar Detox approved.

OLIVES AND OLIVE OIL

When we think of the Mediterranean diet, we immediately think of olives and olive oil. The main reason these little fruits and their oil are so healthy is their fat composition. Olives and olive oils contain mono-unsaturated fatty acids and polyphenols. These polyphenols are a specific type of antioxidant that has antiglycation benefits. The fat in olives and olive oils can lower total cholesterol and LDL levels in the blood, lower blood sugar levels (hooray!), and even lower blood pressure.

Extra-virgin olive oil in particular contains powerful phytonutrients and antioxidants that have an anti-inflammatory effect on the body. It's helpful with cardiovascular health, as it helps repair and protect the heart, which can be damaged by blood sugar fluctuations.

Fruit

As we mentioned earlier, it might seem as if this plan is antifruit, but that's not the case. Fruit is a wonderful source of vitamins, minerals, antioxidants, and fiber. And it also contains a solid amount of sugar. The sugar found in fruit—fructose—raises blood sugar levels rapidly, and even though it's coming from a healthy food source, high levels of blood sugar aren't good for anyone. That said, some fruits are just too good to pass up, even when you're watching your sugar intake. These specific Sugar Detox favorite fruits offer lower fructose levels and low glycemic-index scores, and each has either some added element that helps keep blood sugar levels in check or an amazing anti-aging property that make it worth eating.

Apples

There's a reason for the old saying, "An apple a day keeps the doctor away." You'll notice that apples are one of the main fruits you'll eat on a regular basis on this diet plan, as the first fruit we incorporate back into the meal plan in Week 1. Apples are a great source of fiber (one apple contains about 4 grams), have been tied to lower diabetes risk, contain the super-potent antioxidants, and are low in fructose, while having a low glycemic-index score. All that, in something that you can hold in one hand!

**Sweet *Talk*
BA says:**

"Save on time and money by buying frozen organic fruit—so easy!"

A study published in the *American Journal of Clinical Nutrition* found that people who ate higher amounts of apples tended to have a lower risk of type 2 diabetes, compared with those who didn't eat apples. Score one for the forbidden fruit! Another study, funded by the USDA, found that pectin, the type of fiber in apples, and the polyphenols it contains, could actually improve lipid metabolism and have anti-inflammatory benefits. And here's a third point on the apple scoreboard: A different study from the State University of Rio de Janeiro found that when eating apples as part of a weight-loss plan, women lost more weight and lowered their blood sugar more than did women who consumed an oatmeal-type cookie or pears.

A major component of red apple peel is quercetin, an antioxidant that falls into the flavonoid family and is associated with a decreased risk in type 2 diabetes. Apples also contain another flavonoid called rutin, which has been shown to significantly decrease fasting blood glucose levels and long-term blood glucose levels in people with diabetes. Lastly, this amazing fruit also contains polyphenols called phloretin and phlorizin, which both have major sugar-busting benefits and can inhibit the absorption of glucose and prevent those not-so-pretty AGEs from forming. It's these amazing antioxidants that make apples an all-star fruit on this plan! You can also think of apples as the skin-rejuvenating fruit. All of the apple antioxidants have amazing skin benefits that will be discussed in Chapter 9. So we like to say an apple a day may keep the dermatologist away.

Citrus Fruits

Lemon and lime are used regularly throughout this meal plan, so much so you might start to pucker up a bit. There are many reasons why lemon and lime appear so frequently. First, they can make plain water taste a lot better, therefore you'll drink more of it. A squeeze of either fruit is also like a direct shot of vitamin C. This citrus vitamin helps build collagen, which keeps your skin looking younger and fuller. The acid that comes along with citrus fruit also helps slow down the breakdown of sugar, preventing less sugar spikes (more on that in Chapter 7).

Sweet **Talk**
BA says:
"Even just lemon juice added to water can help with a sweet craving!"

Grapefruit, another approved citrus fruit, has been shown in a study to improve insulin resistance and weight loss. Grapefruits are low on the glycemic index chart and have low levels of fructose; eating grapefruit before a meal also showed a significant reduction in glucose levels after a meal.

Oranges are slightly higher in sugar levels, but the fiber plus the vitamin C levels make them a nice sweet treat to add in Week 3.

Berries

Blackberries, blueberries, raspberries, and strawberries are high in antioxidants, fiber, and vitamin C. The polyphenols that we talked about earlier that are found in apples are also abundant in these tiny fruits; they are major antiglycating antioxidants, meaning they fight the aging process.

Blueberries offer a bonus: In the study that showed eating apples is associated with a lower risk of diabetes, blueberries were demonstrated to have the same impact. The study found that blueberry eaters had a 23 percent lower risk of developing type 2 diabetes than did those who didn't eat any blueberries. While blueberries are higher in fructose levels than we would ideally want, the healthy impact they have on skin and diabetes risk make them worth eating.

Melon

Cantaloupe is allowed starting in Week 2, because although it has a high glycemic index, it's very low in fructose, plus it contains our favorite polyphenols.

Dairy

Dairy, itself, is a type of sugar, so it almost seems like a contradiction to be allowed on the Sugar Detox plan. It's because of the natural sugar, lactose, that we eliminate dairy in the 3-Day Sugar Fix, to help you completely cleanse your system. But dairy done the right way can be a great addition to this plan because it contains protein and fat, which both slow down the absorption of sugar. Dairy done wrong (as will be discussed in Chapter 6), with added sugar or flavorings, should really be thought of as an unhealthy dessert instead of a meal option.

Yogurt, Cottage Cheese, Kefir and Cheese

Plain, unflavored yogurt; cottage cheese; kefir and cheese are great options on the Sugar Detox plan. We only recommend full-fat (yep, you read that right) or low-fat dairy instead of fat-free. The fat is a key part of dairy being allowed, to slow down the absorption of the sugar that these products naturally contain. As mentioned in the fat section on page 56, fat can help curb your appetite by creating a feeling of fullness, triggered by the release of a hormone called cholecystokinin.

YOGURT

Opting for plain flavors and adding your own Sugar Detox–approved spices (think cinnamon!), and later, fruits, is a perfect way to make a plain yogurt into something that not only tastes amazing but has extra benefits. Don't fear the fat here. A large study in Sweden that followed almost twenty thousand women for nine years found that those who increased their whole milk consumption the most, lost on average 9 percent of their body weight. On the other hand, women who increased their low-fat dairy actually gained about 10 percent of their body weight over those 9 years. In addition to the fat, the protein content in these dairy products is also impressive. Greek yogurt is especially high in protein because of the straining process that it undergoes, resulting in a thicker and more satisfying texture, as well as a higher dose of protein. All yogurts and kefirs also contain helpful probiotics that aid in digestion, keep your gut healthy, fight bad bacteria, and have been linked to many other health benefits.

COTTAGE CHEESE AND CHEESE

Other dairy products, such as cottage cheese and cheese, are also good sources of fat and protein, as well as calcium for healthy bones. One ounce of feta cheese in your salad can do a lot of good. It adds a fat content to your meal, which leads to slower absorption of sugar plus a greater level of satiety from the meal itself, meaning that you should be able to feel fuller longer. Crumbled feta or goat cheese tends to be more satisfying than hard cheese, as they are in smaller pieces and have a stronger flavor profile.

The Sugar Detox always recommends that you choose organic dairy products whenever possible.

Dairy Alternatives

Whether it's because you're lactose intolerant or simply don't love dairy, there are plenty of dairy alternatives that are a great substitution or even better than the real deal. The important part of all these dairy alternatives is to make sure they are all unsweetened. That is simply done by reading the ingredients (watch out for such "natural" additives as evaporated cane juice or stevia). Great nondairy options for milk or yogurt are almond milk, coconut milk, and even hemp milk. All unsweetened versions are naturally sugar free and low on the glycemic-index rating. In the last few years they've also become easier to find. Most supermarkets carry nondairy alternatives to milk or yogurt.

Grains

Carbohydrates are often considered the enemy on many diet plans. While some carbs do deserve that title (white bread and white rice should have a mug shot, in our opinion), there are plenty that deserve some recognition and attention. Healthy sources of grain-based carbohydrates add fiber, vitamins, minerals, and more to your diet. Don't fear grains; respect them and eat proper portion sizes. Here are some of our favorite grains. Some of them may be unfamiliar, but give them a try— we promise you'll love the varieties and flavors.

Quinoa

Quinoa is considered an ancient supergrain for many reasons. First, it's a nonanimal source of protein that contains all the essential amino acids that are necessary for your body to build protein molecules.

Quinoa is also a whole grain that hasn't been stripped of all its healthy nutrients by refining, and brings fiber, protein, and healthy fat to the table. With this résumé, quinoa has very little impact on your blood sugar levels, is low on the glycemic-index scale, and is super versatile to cook with (see page 213 for some of our favorite ways to use quinoa!).

Buckwheat

Buckwheat, despite its name, isn't a type of wheat. It's actually a fruit seed (though it doesn't taste sweet), similar to a sunflower seed. These seeds can be eaten plain (great for crunch on yogurt) or can be turned into flour or noodles (soba), kasha, or bran. What's really special about buckwheat is its ability to lower blood glucose levels. A component of buckwheat, D-chiro-inositol, was shown in a study to lower blood glucose levels by 12 to 19 percent. D-chiro-inositol is rarely found in other foods and has been shown to play an important role in glucose metabolism and cell signaling. The most common use of buckwheat is found as buckwheat groats also known as kasha. Kasha can be eaten as any other grain would be and is a delicious side dish or an even better hot breakfast option. Buckwheat can also be made into soba noodle. These noodles contain protein and fiber, helping slow down sugar absorption, and are low on the glycemic index, which is why this option is considered a Sugar Detox all-star. Buckwheat groats are the hulled seeds of the buckwheat plant. These crunchy seeds are mild in flavor but add a great texture to yogurt for a cereal alternative.

> **Sweet Talk**
> **Dr. F says:**
> *"The niacin in whole grains gives skin a natural, rosy glow."*

Other Whole Grains

Other amazing healthy grains include oatmeal, amaranth, brown rice, barley, and bulgur. All of these grains are low-glycemic-index foods that contain fiber. Oatmeal is best known for its heart-health benefits, due to the soluble fiber it contains. It's soluble fiber that keeps you fuller longer and reduces bad cholesterol.

Pasta

Most pastas tend to be high in sugar, but in the last few years there has been a surge in the market for healthier pasta options. Big-name brands, such as Barilla, are now making protein-enriched or whole-grain pastas that are easy to find and taste really good. We'll talk more in the next chapter about why we avoid plain pasta, but whole-grain pasta or protein-enriched pastas in proper servings are a great addition to your diet. (You'll be adding pasta back in during Week 3!)

Beverages

You might have already noticed that throughout the program we are constantly advising you to drink—water, green tea, herbal tea, coffee, and even wine! (A Sugar Detox disclaimer: If you do not drink alcohol or are underage, then obviously alcohol should be avoided completely.) Your number one beverage priority should always be water.

Water

We all know that it's necessary for your body's essential functioning, but water is more than a hydration tool. In a study published in *Diabetes Care*, the journal for the American Diabetes Association, researchers linked low water intake with high blood sugar. Adults who drank only about two glasses of water daily (roughly half a liter) were more likely to have high blood sugar. The connection here could be a hormone called vasopressin, which helps regulate water retention. When you are dehydrated, vasopressin levels increase to alert your kidneys to conserve water, but research also suggests a relationship between high levels of vasopressin and elevated blood sugar. While further studies are still necessary to prove this connection completely, water is clearly an important factor in overall health. Your skin is also one of the first places where you can see dehydration. Dehydrated skin looks older and more wrinkled, and has less elasticity—getting thirsty yet?

Red Wine

You might be relieved to find that red wine is included in the diet plan of the Sugar Detox. The reason isn't that we want everyone a little tipsy; it's that red wine contains several powerful antioxidants, including one called resveratrol. This is a type of polyphenol that's considered the big shot in the antioxidant world. Resveratrol has been linked to everything from lowering blood sugar and preventing damage to blood vessels, to lowering LDL cholesterol and increased longevity.

Resveratrol in red wine comes from the grape skins that are used to make wine. Red wine is fermented with the skins for longer than the process with white wine, making red wine a more powerful source. Eating grapes can also provide you with resveratrol, so if you don't drink already, there is no reason to begin; just add grapes during Week 3, watching your portion size.

Research has shown some promising results on resveratrol. It is now confirmed that dietary resveratrol mimics the benefits of extremely difficult caloric restriction, including improving cardiovascular health and reducing age-related illnesses. Resveratrol has also been shown to help with glucose metabolism and improve insulin sensitivity. At present, there is much debate about resveratrol and studies are ongoing to validate the numerous health claims being made about this antioxidant superstar. The biggest question seems to be, does resveratrol really enhance longevity? Only time will tell. But for now, we think it's reasonable to suggest that you enjoy that occasional glass of red wine in the evening, and who knows, it may even been good for you. We'll say "cheers" to that!

Green Tea

You'll notice that another color keeps popping up here, too. And it's green—as in green tea. Green tea has long been acclaimed for its health benefits, largely due to its high content of antioxidants called flavonoids. In green tea, these flavonoids are a specific type called catechins, which are incredibly powerful—even more so than vitamins C and E in preventing oxidative damage to cells—and have been linked to a reduced risk of many different types of cancers. People who regularly consume green, black, and oolong teas are also at a reduced risk for heart disease, as these beverages help prevent oxidation of LDL cholesterol, raise HDL cholesterol, and improve artery function. A large study in Europe found a connection with tea drinkers and a reduced risk of diabetes, concluding that people who drank at least four cups of tea per day might have up to a 16 percent lower risk of developing diabetes than did non–tea drinkers. Green tea polyphenols have also been shown to have antiglycation properties. Studies have confirmed that ingestion of green tea extract effectively inhibited AGE accumulation that's associated with aging.

Sweet Talk

Dr. F says:

"When you brew green tea, don't throw out the tea bags. Cool them down in the fridge and use them as a compress on the under-eye area."

Not only is green tea healthy, but it can also help you lose weight. In a study published in the *American Journal of Clinical Nutrition*, researchers found that daily consumption of tea with high levels of catechins (i.e., green tea) can reduce body fat. Another study showed that green tea helped increase feeling of satiety and fullness after a meal, so people were more likely to consume fewer calories and feel more satisfied with what they ate. We'll drink to that!

Herbs and Spices

When you begin using our recipes, you'll become very quickly familiar with the herb and spice aisle at your local market. There are a few reasons for this. First, herbs and spices are a great way to add tons of flavor to food without adding any sodium, sugar, or extra calories. Second, multiple studies have shown that certain herbs and spices can have a major impact on health, affecting everything from inflammation to blood sugar levels to preventing the glycation process.

Let's review what the glycation process is—it's when sugar in the blood attaches to your body's proteins, such as collagen and elastin, and causes them to become stiff, rigid, and unable to be repaired. This leaves your skin looking older and more wrinkled. Certain spices, including ginger, cinnamon, allspice, and cloves, are the most potent when it comes to preventing glycation. In addition, herbs such as sage, marjoram, tarragon, and rose-mary were also found to be effective in preventing glycation. A study published in the *Journal of Medic-inal Foods* reinforces this notion. It found a strong cor-relation between the antioxidant content of common herbs and spices and their ability to prevent glycation and formation of dreaded AGEs.

> **Sweet *Talk***
> **Dr. F says:**
> *"Choose more colorful foods—they contain more antioxidants."*

Cinnamon

Cinnamon is an especially favorite spice in the Sugar Detox plan, as it can help the body to become more sensitive to insulin, basically telling cells to wake up and smell the insulin and get to work putting away sugar properly. In addition, researchers in Pakistan (cinnamon's home-land) found that people with type 2 diabetes who consumed cinnamon saw their blood glucose levels drop by almost 30 percent.

Turmeric

Turmeric, a beautiful bright yellow spice that is a relative of ginger, is commonly used in Indian cuisine (it's what gives tandoori-style foods and curries their beautiful color). Turmeric has been shown in numer-ous and promising studies to have major health benefits: It can help prevent carcinogens from occurring on barbecued, broiled, or fried meats; and it also has been shown that curcumin, the main active component in turmeric, can inhibit growth and progression of many cancers. It is also hypothesized that India has such low rate of Alzheimer's disease because of the large amount of turmeric consumed in that country. (Studies have shown that turmeric's power is enhanced when you add freshly ground black pepper, when cooking with turmeric.)

All-Star Food List

Kale
Broccoli
Eggs
Wild salmon
Lentils
Pistachios
Chia seeds
Apples
Blueberries
Oatmeal
Soba noodles
Greek yogurt
Green tea
Dark chocolate

Herbs and spices can also be beneficial when used in teas. There are so many amazing brands of teas that have wonderful flavors that allow you to drink up all the benefits of herbs and spices.

All herbs and spices are amazing sources of antioxidants and all can be beneficial to total health; we encourage you to get spicy and try them out!

Chocolate

By Week 3 of the plan, dark chocolate has never looked so good. Dark chocolate, with a high cacao content of more than 65 percent, has amazing health benefits and that's why it's the number one (and only) approved sweet treat on the Sugar Detox. Dark chocolate comes with a stellar résumé: It contains lots of antioxidants, including flavonoids (just like apples), that protect cells from free radicals and oxidative stress. Scientific studies have shown that the flavonoids in dark chocolate can reduce blood pressure by producing nitric oxide, which relaxes blood vessels, making it easier for blood to flow. Cacao, the main ingredient in dark chocolate, lowers LDL cholesterol by blocking intestinal absorption of cholesterol. A study published in the *British Medical Journal,* showed that dark chocolate could even be considered a cheap intervention strategy for a population with a high risk of cardiovascular disease. All of these results were for dark chocolate with a high content of cacao, so if you were thinking about munching down on your favorite candy bar—forget about it. That's still a no-no in our book, because most regular candy bars contain tons of added sugar and normally don't use a high-quality dark chocolate.

Another positive effect of the dark stuff is that it can help improve your mood. Sometimes, following a diet (even if it's as awesome as this one) can make you a little cranky. Fortunately, by Week 3, you'll have no excuse to scowl anymore. Dark chocolate can stimulate the production of chemicals in your brain called endorphins that bring on the feeling of pleasure. It also contains serotonin, which acts as a natural antidepressant. The flavonoids in dark chocolate may also have some skin benefits. In a study comparing dark chocolate with high flavanol (a type of flavonoid) levels with regular chocolate that has low flavanol levels, those who ate dark chocolate daily for three months showed significant protection from UV light. Now we don't suggest you give up your sunscreen for chocolate just yet, but these results do suggest chocolate may do more than just satisfy your sweet tooth.

While dark chocolate isn't specifically linked to helping lower blood sugar, it naturally contains fat resulting in a slower absorption of the sugars it contains. Chocolate might help you stay thin, too. A study published in the *Archives of Internal Medicine* showed that people who enjoyed chocolate a few times a week had a lower body-mass index (BMI) than those who indulged less often. This could possibly be because of an antioxidant called epicatechins that can potentially rev your metabolism. All the more reason why chocolate gets our approval as a portioned-controlled treat!

New Foods to Try and How to Eat Them

Some of the foods we mention may be new to you. Here at Sugar Detox central, we're all about encouraging new, healthy foods to try. Here's a quick chart outlining the benefits of some of our favorites, with suggestions for easy ways to work them into your diet.

FOOD	WHY	HOW TO EAT
Chia seeds	These tiny poppylike seeds contain mega-doses of omega 3-fatty acids and tons of fiber.	Make Chia Pudding (page 179) or simply sprinkle the seeds on top of yogurt for a yummy crunch.
Hemp seeds	These nutty-tasting seeds are a complete vegetarian source of protein, while also containing fiber and omega-3s.	Use on top of salads or oatmeal, in smoothies or pancakes (sprinkle into our pancakes, page 179), or eat raw.
Flaxseeds	These brown seeds contain huge amounts of alpha-linolenic acid, a type of omega-3 fatty acid.	Sprinkle ground seeds into parfaits or oatmeal, use the oil in smoothies or add to salad dressings.
Kelp	Kelp is rich in B vitamins, as well as vitamin C and E, which are strong antioxidants.	Kelp noodles are great in stir-fries and soups, and even mixed into salads.
Coconut butter and oil	Coconut butter and oil contain medium-chain fatty acids that can be used for energy instead of fat storage.	Spread coconut butter on top of Cottage Cheese–Oatmeal Pancakes (page 179) or crackers; use coconut oil for sautéing and cooking.
Kale chips	Kale chips are made from the iron-rich green, which contains tons of antioxidants and fiber.	Kale chips can be made or purchased, and are a great crunchy way to get in your leafy greens.

6

What *Not* to Eat

Now that we've focused on the positive part of the diet, all the great foods that should be eaten regularly—we do need to alert you to some others that are counterproductive and could really sabotage your Sugar Detox. This chapter tells you why you need to break up with some of your favorites.

SWEET SUCCESS
Lance

"I have been overweight for years and suffer with joint pains, especially in my ankles and knees almost every day. I am on my feet all day at work, so by the end of the day it can be pretty painful. Once I started the diet, it was dramatic how fast I started feeling better. My joint pains went away in just a couple days, and I stuck to the plan and lost 12 pounds in four weeks. When I cheat, and I do on occasion, my joint pain comes back almost immediately. I was hooked on Diet Coke before I started this diet and found it really easy to put that behind me. Now I only drink healthy drinks, mostly water with lime. I am actually down 25 pounds now and I feel great. I'm not hungry and have lots of energy and no joint pains."

White Flour

We discussed in Chapter 3 the refining process that turns a grain into a sugary mess. When the bran and the germ are stripped from wheat, what remains is a simple carbohydrate that's rapidly absorbed by your body. With this quick absorption also comes a tendency to eat more, because you don't have the same feeling of fullness that you would if you ate something containing fiber or protein. Wheat also has a type of carbohydrate called amylopectin A. This carbohydrate is extra potent when it's in white flour, because the lack of fiber causes it to convert more easily to blood sugar than does just about any other carbohydrate. In addition, white flour has a very high glycemic-index rating. A 2004 research study published in the journal *Lancet* showed that a high-glycemic diet sends the body right into fat storage mode, instead of those calories being used for muscle burning.

Sweet *Talk*

Dr. F says:

"As it turns out, those old wives' tales were right all along: Some foods do trigger acne breakouts!"

Modern white flour (as compared to the flour our ancestors used to eat) contains a type of protein called gliadin. Gliadin causes a feel-good effect in the brain and increases people's appetite—one of the reasons that white flour foods, such as pasta, are high on the list of comfort foods.

Another favorite comfort food that's more foe than friend is the ubiquitous bagel. These days, a plain, average-size bagel is the equivalent in calories and sugar of five slices of white bread and sends your system into a sugar overload . . . only setting you up to crash afterward and wanting to reach for another unhealthy option. Bottom line: Stick to the whole grains and keep your portion sizes small.

AVOID | All refined white carbs (most processed/packaged foods), especially white pasta, bagels, biscuits, white wraps, and white bread.

White Rice

White rice seems so harmless, yet it's like sugar in a bowl. The refining process that rice goes through takes a whole rice grain and turns it into just the endosperm, an easily digestible, fiberless starch. While the glycemic index of rice does vary based on the cooking time and the rice variety, all forms of white rice are high on the glycemic-index scale and will cause a sugar spike when eaten. Starchy foods without fiber also tend to be eaten in bigger portions, because you don't feel as full from them without the fiber to slow down their digestion. Recent studies have shown that eating white rice can raise blood sugar significantly, especially eaten often or in large quantities. One study specifically showed an 11 percent increase in diabetes risk with each daily serving of white rice. Opt instead for brown rice or other high-fiber grains, such as quinoa.

White rice. **AVOID**

Starchy Vegetables

It seems so wrong to put any vegetable on the "avoid" list, but the truth is that some of these veggies are starches in disguise. Such vegetables as corn, potatoes and sweet potatoes, winter squash (e.g., butternut and pumpkin), and beets are high in dietary starches and also have high GI values (as we've learned, that means when you eat them, your blood sugar levels rise too quickly). That said, these vegetables do contain some health benefits from the vitamins and minerals they contain and are certainly better options than desserts, so don't forgo squash in favor of cake. But if you want the best and quickest results from this plan, these veggies just don't make the cut.

Corn, potatoes, sweet potatoes, winter squash, and beets. **AVOID**

High-GI Fruit

As with starchy vegetables, it seems to go against what we know of healthy eating to say to avoid bananas, pineapple, and watermelon. While these fruits have tons of health benefits, they are all high in sugar and we think it's best for you to avoid them. We'd much rather you opt for some lower-sugar fruits that will have less of an impact on your blood sugar levels and therefore won't cause any insulin imbalance. With so many other healthy fruit options, we don't even think you'll miss these. Even a fruit that's high in sugar can start your cravings again, so pick up an apple or some berries instead!

AVOID | Bananas, pineapple, and watermelon.

Dried Fruit

Fruit is dried so it can last longer and be portable, allowing you to take it with you without spoilage. This is great if you're an extreme hiker and can carry only some foods with you and need instant energy on the go. But for most of us, dried fruit shouldn't be a go-to snack. The drying process removes water from the fruit, making the fruit a more condensed version of its prior self with more sugar. More often than not, dried fruits, such as dried cranberries, have added sugars in them as well, increasing the jump in your blood sugar even more quickly. Dried fruit does contain healthy vitamins and minerals and some fiber, but the sugar content tends to outweigh the health benefits here. While eating dried fruit is healthier than snacking on processed candy, it still sends your blood sugar for a ride. There's a reason why these snacks are called "nature's candy."

AVOID | All dried fruits, especially dates, cranberries, raisins, and prunes.

Sweetened Dairy Products

Dairy is a kind of sugar on its own, but it's allowed starting in the first week because its protein content slows the absorption of that sugar. As noted in Chapter 5, all the dairy products we recommend are unsweetened: Choose only cottage cheese, cheese, milk, yogurt, or nondairy substitutes that have no added sugars.

Many soy and other dairy-alternative milks contain added sugars and are to be avoided; likewise, flavored dairy products such as chocolate milk.

The flavored yogurts you find filling the refrigerated shelves in the supermarkets (and make that double or maybe even triple for frozen yogurt!) are basically just sugary versions of what yogurt should really be like. This includes all those seemingly plain yogurts that have fruit on the bottom; yep, they're loaded with sugar, too (if you're ever in doubt, just check the ingredients list). If you don't really like plain yogurt, you can jazz it up yourself by adding some cinnamon, fresh berries, and a sprinkle of slivered almonds. You won't miss all that unnecessary sugar at all!

Sweetened milk or milk substitutes, flavored yogurts, flavored cottage cheese. | **AVOID**

Juice

Nothing hits your bloodstream quicker than fruit juice. Because juice has no protein or fiber, it's a super quick way to spike your blood sugar levels. Fruit juice is unnecessary and we prefer that you eat a piece of fruit so as to get the chew factor (which is more satisfying), plus the fiber that will help delay the sugar rush. Vegetable juices are a slightly better option, even more so if they are a green vegetable juice. But more often than not, they end up a mix of some greens plus tons of fruit to make them taste better, so these really aren't a good option. If fresh green juices are of interest, opt for only one fruit per juice and ideally use only an apple. It will add sweetness without lots of sugar and can count as your apple serving for the day. Even the commercial juice brands that claim to have less sugar in them still cause a major sugar rush. Flavor water instead in a pitcher—just add cucumber or lemon slices and chill. Delicious, hydrating, and no sugar!

AVOID

Fruit juice, vegetable juices with extra fruit.

Sodas

Sodas, be they diet or regular, are completely off limits in the Sugar Detox plan. Regular soda has no nutritional value; it is basically a bunch of chemicals and artificial colors plus a steady stream of liquid sugar in a large cup with a straw. It is shouldn't be included in any healthy diet.

As we discussed earlier, there is no evidence that artificial sweeteners are safe to consume and new evidence suggests that they are just as bad as real sugar when it comes to insulin and blood sugar levels. So suffice it to say that we insist that you avoid all artificial sweeteners. *This means no diet soda!* A study published in the *American Journal of Clinical Nutrition* found that people who ate a healthy diet rich in fresh fruits and vegetables but also drank diet soda were at a greater risk of developing metabolic syndrome than were those who didn't. Another long-term study found that diet soda drinkers' waistlines expanded by 70 percent more than occurred among nondrinkers over a ten-year period. Those who drank more than two diet sodas a day were almost five times more likely to gain weight than were those who didn't.

Although you may think that diet soda will help your sugar cravings, it actually does the opposite: Drinking or consuming artificial sweeteners messes with your palate. They are much sweeter—some as much as 700 percent as sweet!—than regular sugar and cause an imbalance in your taste bud sensitivity that prevents you from perceiving what normal sweetness taste likes. This makes you need more sugar, fake or real, to be satisfied with the sweet stuff.

By the end of the 3-Day Sugar Fix, you might start to taste the natural sugars in food that you haven't been able to taste in years. You'll find that you'll discover the natural sweetness in so many unexpected foods—even almonds are sweet—when you take a break from all the fake stuff and taste what a natural healthy sugar option is like.

Soda, diet sodas, artificial sweeteners of any kind. **AVOID**

7

How to Eat

The main goal of the Sugar Detox is to change the way you eat so you are consuming less sugar and instead eating delicious foods with more fiber, antioxidants, and overall nutrients. Once you get the hang of this, you'll feel more satiated, won't have those midday slumps or crashes, and won't be craving sugar at every turn. For this to happen, a few things need to occur. First, you need to know what to eat (Chapter 5); then what to avoid (Chapter 6); and finally, how foods interact, so as to optimize your results. That's what's special about this chapter: We discuss when, how, and which foods to eat together. Something as simple as making sure you have protein or fat with your meals can make a huge difference with how your body digests what you're eating!

When you arrive at a restaurant, do you start filling up on the bread-basket before your food is even served? Do you ever skip breakfast and then find yourself overeating later in the day? What about water—are you dehydrated right now? All of these are common mistakes we all make. Here are our suggestions for avoiding these blunders. Follow them and you'll find that you will lose weight more quickly and start feeling and looking better faster.

Eat Breakfast Every Morning

Yep, you've heard it before and you're hearing it here, too. Breakfast is important for many reasons, particularly because it wakes up your

"I was a little nervous before I started the Sugar Detox. I wasn't sure exactly how my body would react to the withdrawal of not only processed and/or refined sugar, but also to natural sugar as well. I was pleasantly surprised by how easy it was to let it all go! In the first three days I made significant changes to my diet, based on the plan, and quickly came to realize that not only could I live without all that sugar (especially the artificial sweeteners), but I actually enjoyed how my coffee and food tasted without it. Feasting on mostly veggies and lean meat, I immediately felt less bloated, had brighter skin, and was much more alert. I ended up losing 4 pounds after the first few days. In the subsequent weeks, I looked forward to adding some fruit and cheese on occasion, and also some high-fiber crackers as suggested. My intense sugar cravings, however, had diminished a great deal. I also felt less hungry and more satisfied at each meal. I highly recommend this plan to help change your body and your life."

metabolism after you have basically fasted all night while you slept. Breakfast allows you to refuel after hours of not eating, increasing your total energy level. Studies have shown that people who skip their morning meal tend to suffer from mood issues, impaired memory, and low energy. These breakfast skippers are also more likely to gain weight, for two reasons: (1) prolonged fasting increases the body's insulin response; leading to fat storage and weight gain; and (2) skipping breakfast sets you up to overeat for the rest of the day. Nixing breakfast can trigger poor food choices, such as your giving in to the lure of the snack array in a vending machine or including a doughnut with that cup of coffee. As if that wasn't enough reason to have a bite when you wake up, research has shown that people who consistently eat breakfast have a reduced risk of type 2 diabetes. A 2012 study, published in the *American Journal of Clinical Nutrition*, which followed almost thirty thousand men found that those who skipped breakfast on a regular basis had over a 20 percent higher risk of developing diabetes than did those who ate their morning meal. The exact mechanism of why this is the case isn't precisely clear, but it's been suggested that breakfast can help stabilize blood sugar throughout the day.

Snack Attack

While it might seem as if you never get a break from eating when you follow the Sugar Detox schedule that includes snack breaks, consistent snacking of approved foods is what helps this diet work. First of all, eating modest amounts frequently will stabilize your blood sugar, because you're not allowing it to drop too drastically or to rise too sharply throughout the day. The other advantage to snacking is that by the time you get to your next meal, you aren't starving. The last thing we want you to do is to make poor food choices or wolf down even a healthy meal because you're so hungry. This tip allows you to think rationally and make better choices. Just think: If you were to arrive at a restaurant for dinner for an eight PM reservation and you hadn't eaten anything since one PM, would you have the patience to read the menu thoroughly to find something that really meets your needs? Even if you're eating at home, how many times do you find yourself so hungry that you graze while waiting for your meal to be ready? We've all been there. By eating Sugar Detox–approved snacks between meals, you set yourself up for success at every meal.

Get Puckered

Ever just ignore that lemon that comes with your glass of water when you eat out? Don't skip it. Lemon, lime, and even vinegar are all beneficial to help slow down digestion. Lemon and limes contain plenty of polyphenols, the stellar antioxidants that neutralize free radicals and prevent those pesky AGEs from forming. Because lemons and limes are very low on the glycemic-index rating and contain barely any fructose, they're allowed even in the 3-Day Sugar Fix. They are both loaded with vitamin C as well, which is a natural collagen booster.

Vinegar is not just a tangy condiment, either. An interesting study performed in Sweden found that eating a meal that included vinegar reduced spikes in blood sugar and insulin after the meal and also increased feelings of fullness. This reaction is likely due to vinegar's acetic acid, which slows down digestion, thereby slowing down sugar absorption. The flavor of vinegar is also very satisfying and can result in fewer calories being consumed if this condiment is included in a meal. Dip some crudités in red wine vinegar; use our vinaigrette (page 178) as a salad dressing or mix it with avocado as a spread. However you consume these small additions to your flavor palette, they can have a big and beneficial impact on your body—so pucker up!

Drink Up

Water is key in any healthy lifestyle. The fabulous H_2O makes up 60 percent of your body weight (and 70 percent of your brain) and every system in your body depends on it. Water is necessary for everything from flushing out toxins to delivering nutrients to cells. And a study funded by the Institute for Public Health and Water Research found that drinking water before each meal can promote weight loss, by creating a feeling of fullness. It's also common to confuse thirst or dehydration with hunger; when our thirst is satisfied, we can be more in touch with our true hunger, allowing us to pay more attention to what's on our plate instead of overeating or eating past satiety.

Hydration also affects your skin quality and appearance. Dehydrated skin loses its elasticity, or "snap," leading to a more aged appearance. When doctors want to check how hydrated a patient is, they assess the individual's skin to determine whether he or she is consuming enough water.

Water also boosts energy levels. Even mild dehydration can drain your energy and make you tired. Instead of reaching for that cup of cof-

Sweet Talk
BA says:

"If you sit at a desk all day, set a liter bottle of water on it and try to finish it before you leave at the end of the day—that way you'll know that you're getting hydrated."

fee or a sweet snack when you're tired, consider having an extra glass of water instead, to get you going.

Eat Protein First

Just as pairing wine with meals brings out the flavor, pairing certain foods together can have some great benefits. One of the most important meal pairings is making sure that when you consume your carbohydrates or sugar, it's eaten with some protein. There are a few important reasons for this.

First, protein is satisfying. Regardless of its source, protein makes you feel fuller, leading you to consume fewer total calories during the meal. Also, starting each meal with a lean source of protein (see page 53) prevents any major sugar spike. Instead, your body's energy is focused on breaking down protein into amino acids that can help your body control blood sugar. Then, by eating the rest of a meal that is comprised predominately of low-glycemic-index and low-fructose foods, you will avoid sugar spikes and your body will remain in a constant stable place.

Even if you were to eat a non-approved food (how could you!), you will have less of a reaction to it if it is consumed with some protein. Consider this: If you haven't eaten in more than three hours and the first bite of food you take is a piece of fruit, instead of your system being able to break down the fruit and utilize the best parts of it—its antioxidants, fiber, vitamin C, and more—your body instead says "Feed me" and goes for the sugar. As the fruit contains no protein that could slow down the absorption, that sugar is swept up into your bloodstream super fast, signaling your pancreas to release insulin to help absorb it, thereby telling your body to convert the extra sugar to fat. Fruit is not the enemy here; it's sugar. Regardless of the form it is in when it enters an empty stomach, sugar converts too quickly into fat, can glycate collagen structures, and lead to inflammation. All of this can be stopped by your combining your approved sweets with protein foods, such as having some eggs in the morning prior to your small bowl of mixed berries, or eating some nuts or peanut butter with your apple as a snack.

Have Some Fat with Each Meal

Similar to, "It takes money to make money," we believe it takes fat to lose fat. Consuming the right kind of fat with meals actually prevents blood sugar spikes.

There are two reasons why we require you to have a minimum of at least three healthy fats a day. First, as discussed in Chapter 3, fat has some amazing benefits—everything from heart health to healthy skin. Second, fat slows down gastric emptying. That basically means that fat causes the transportation of food from your stomach to intestine to slow down (think of it as increasing the traffic on your food high-way). This isn't a bad thing, as it prevents quick absorption of sugar into your bloodstream. A study published in the *Journal of Clinical Endocrinology Metabolism* showed that the ingestion of fat prior to eating a carbohydrate-heavy meal slowed the absorption of sugar and reduced blood sugar spikes.

Take a look at your plate at each meal and make sure that you're getting some healthy fat with whatever you're eating. Even if you're just having a plain Greek yogurt, sprinkle some flaxseeds into it, add a few slices of avocado to your open-faced multigrain sandwich, toss a few olives into your salad . . . your options are endless!

Let Water Cook for You

As discussed on page 42, how you prepare your food counts, too. Although grilled, fried, and roasted foods taste yummy, the AGEs formed in such browning practices wreak havoc in your body and on your skin.

Here again, water comes to the rescue: Your best bet is to poach, boil, or steam your food. In Chapter 13 we offer recipes that show easy ways to incorporate these healthy methods to produce tasty snacks and meals. And guess what? We also introduce you to roasting or broiling methods that are super delicious, healthy, and user friendly, too, to help you stay motivated to stay with the Sugar Detox program.

Spice It Up

Having just warned you off browning foods, we have a tip for you: If you can't poach, boil, or steam your protein options, then make sure you cook with plenty of herbs and spices, to help offset or even prevent the AGEs created by grilling, frying, and roasting from forming. And if you find your poached, boiled, or steamed foods bland, herbs and spices are great additions to punch up the flavor. Try adding herbs, such as rosemary and thyme, to salads, veggies, and even whole wheat pasta. Spices are a nifty addition to beverages, too: Add ground cinnamon or ginger to your tea or coffee and it will make you forget about the sugar you might be missing. See page 8 for a list of recommended herbs and spices to get you going.

Nutty Buddy

On this plan, your new best friends are nuts. Nuts contain nutrients and phytochemicals and are full of good fats. People who eat lots of nuts have less inflammation and oxidative stress and are less likely to develop insulin resistance. Nuts also lower cholesterol levels and may protect diabetics from cardiovascular disease. On the Sugar Detox plan, you can use nuts as a snack and incorporate them into your cooked foods. In other words, just go nuts!

We suggest you keep a bag of your favorite nuts handy. Put them in your desk drawer at work so you can grab a handful for a snack. And check out Chapter 13 to see how to incorporate nuts into delicious meals and snacks, such as our Pistachio Pesto (page 211) or Sweetish Nuts (page 216)! Just watch your portions; while we are nut lovers, too many nuts can add calories, so aim for one serving a day, or two if you find yourself extra hungry!

Go Whole

It may seem strange to not be throwing out the yolk when making your breakfast eggs in the morning or not pouring that milk that's slight blue into your coffee, but in our Sugar Detox, we promote going whole. That's right, whole eggs and full or low-fat dairy products. No more fat-free for you! You already know from previous chapters that you needn't fear fat anymore, and that the hormone cholecystokinin, released when fat is consumed, causes the feeling of fullness. So those whole eggs and dairy products help you feel more satisfied.

Egg yolks have long been vilified, starting with the low-fat craze. It is true that egg yolks contain some fat and cholesterol, but they are still safe to eat. Dietary cholesterol does not lead to an increase in your blood cholesterol levels. Whole eggs also contain many amazing nutrients that are key to good health. For example, they are an amazing source of choline, an essential nutrient for brain functioning, as well as other important B vitamins.

Because dairy contains natural sugars, the fat in whole-milk dairy products will help delay that sugar absorption from happening too quickly. Do a taste test, too. How much more do you like whole-milk dairy products than those that are fat-free? Between the product's mouthfeel and how satisfying it is, we think there is no reason not to go whole here!

Drink and Be Merry

We made an executive decision early on that a diet without drinking was like a party without music. Boring! We know that you might prefer to abstain completely and we are completely supportive of that decision. But if you enjoy relaxing in the evening with an alcoholic beverage in hand, we are giving you the green light—as long as you follow the rules. First, beer is off the list because it's full of sugar—but red wine gets the thumbs-up because it's full of antioxidants that are good for you. Second, drinking must be done in moderation. Yes, the days of drinking a bottle of wine between the two of you every night are over. That's what we mean by moderation.

One of the things that we have been told by those who have followed our program over the long term is that they can no longer overindulge in alcoholic beverages without grave consequences, such as bad hang-overs. We suspect that all of this clean living and eating just lowers your tolerance for alcoholic beverages. And that's a good thing. Drinking al-cohol in moderation also helps keep your eating more honest: When you drink, your inhibitions go down slightly and it makes you more will-ing to take an extra bite of dessert or try those French fries or the bread on the table. While none of these are that bad on their own, they add up throughout a meal, and before you know it, your dinner went from Sugar Detox to disaster.

Part Three

THE Plan

8

Detoxing Your Diet,
Week by Week

Now that you know all the science and have all the tools, it's time to jump into the weekly plans. If you haven't yet done the 3-Day Sugar Fix, you'll want to start with that. Remember, you're removing a significant toxin from your diet, so you may have feelings of withdrawal: fatigue, fogginess, headaches, and intense cravings. Yes, they are unpleasant—but they are signs that your body is ridding itself of toxins and getting ready for a whole new healthy existence, and you'll feel terrific in a few days once your body is free of all that extra sugar you have been carrying around in your system.

As we mentioned earlier, our weekly plans build on our 3-Day Plan, while including additional approved foods as directed each week. We include sample menus to give you some idea of how to plan your meals around each week's selections, and provide a day-by-day guide to 31 days' worth of suggested meals and snacks in Appendix A, pages 223–231. You will notice that we occasionally recommend approved-brand products, such as yogurt or pasta; please see Appendix B, pages 233–239, for a list of commercially packaged goods that happily fit within the parameters of the Sugar Detox.

Vegetarians and Vegans, Take Note

Both vegetarians and vegans can follow the Sugar Detox. Tofu can re-place any meat or egg products for any meal. Legumes, such as beans, can also serve as your protein substitute; just watch your por-tion sizes. Unsweetened almond, coconut, or soymilk or yogurts can be used as a dairy substitute. Just read the ingredients to make sure no sugars, such as evaporated cane syrup, are listed.

3-Day Sugar Fix Approved Foods

- 1 cup of unsweetened black coffee per day
- Unsweetened green and/or herbal tea, in unlimited amounts
- Minimum 64 ounces of water (sparkling water or club soda is okay) daily
- Protein: lean red meat, pork, chicken, turkey, fish, shellfish, eggs, tofu, or legumes (see box above for vegetarian/vegan options; see serving sizes for protein on page 7)
- Veggies: approved veggies (see page 7) in unlimited amounts
- Fruits: lemon or lime, for drinks or cooking
- Nuts: a 1-ounce serving of nuts (see page 7) may be eaten twice daily as a snack.
- Condiments and cooking oil: red wine vinegar, balsamic vinegar, or apple cider vinegar; and olive oil, coconut oil, or butter for cooking
- Herbs and spices: unlimited amounts

No-No's

- Artificial sweeteners of any kind—and that includes diet drinks
- Alcohol
- Dairy (except a little butter for cooking)
- Wheat or other starches, such as pasta, cereal, rice, quinoa, and so on
- Added sugar of any kind
- Fruit (except lemon or lime for drinks or for cooking)

Cooking Techniques
- Sauté
- Stir-fry
- Poach
- Steam
- Boil

Remember to use only the oils on the approved list!

WEEK 1 Continue Sugar Free . . . But You Get Wine and Cheese!

The first week following the 3-day Sugar Fix is the most important week of the plan, as this is when you will start seeing some great changes in how you're feeling. The withdrawal symptoms you may have experienced during the first three days should have subsided, while your energy will start increasing. During this week, you will continue to abstain from sugar in general but slowly allow some natural sugar back into your diet (hello, wine and cheese) along with some variations from eating the same foods each day. During this week, you will be eating no starches except high-fiber crackers, and an apple a day, Why apples? Apples are a low-sugar fruit with lots of fiber. They also contain antioxidants that inhibit glycation.

Week 1 Approved Foods
- 2 cups of unsweetened coffee per day max, plus 2 tablespoons of 2% milk if desired
- Unsweetened green and/or herbal tea, in unlimited amounts
- Minimum 64 ounces of water (sodium-free sparkling water or club soda is okay) daily
- Protein: lean red meat, pork, chicken, turkey, fish, shellfish, eggs, tofu, or legumes (see box on page 94 for vegetarian/vegan options; see serving sizes for protein on page 7)
- Dairy: 1 serving per day (1 ounce of cheese, 5 ounces of yogurt, or ½ cup of cottage cheese, ½ cup of 2% or whole milk or milk alternative per day) of the following dairy or dairy alternatives, in addition to the optional splash in coffee:

- o Almond milk (see approved-brands list, page 236)
- o American cheese
- o Cheddar cheese
- o Cottage cheese (low-fat)
- o Feta cheese
- o Greek yogurt (see approved-brands list, page 239)
- o Milk (2% or whole)
- o Mozzarella cheese
- o Parmesan cheese
- o Provolone cheese
- o Ricotta cheese (part skim)
- o Soy milk (see approved-brands list, page 236)
- o String cheese

- Veggies: approved veggies (see page 7) in unlimited amounts, plus any of the following:
  - o Carrots (raw)
  - o Onions (raw)
  - o Spaghetti squash
  - o Summer squash
  - o Snow peas
  - o Tomatoes

- Fruits: 1 medium-size apple per day; plus lemon or lime, for drinks or cooking
- Nuts: a 1-ounce serving of nuts (see page 7) may be eaten up to twice daily as an additional snack.
- Seeds: a 1-ounce serving of sunflower seeds may be eaten up to twice daily as an additional snack
- Fat: minimum 3 servings (from oils, olives, avocados, nuts, or seeds)
- Starch: 1 serving of approved-brand high-fiber crackers (2 crackers unless otherwise noted as a serving on the product label; (see approved-brands list, page 233)

- Alcohol: 1 glass (5 fluid ounces) of red wine only, three times per week max
- Condiments and cooking oil: red wine vinegar, balsamic or apple cider vinegar and olive oil, coconut oil or butter for cooking
- Herbs and spices: unlimited amounts

Cooking Techniques
- Sauté
- Steam
- Stir-fry
- Boil
- Poach

Remember to use only the oils on the approved list!

Week 1 Sample Daily Menu
See Chapter 13 or Recipe Index (page 257) for asterisked (*) recipes; if double-asterisked (**), see Appendix B for approved brands.

BREAKFAST: Greek yogurt** with 2 tablespoons of ground flaxseeds and 1 tablespoon of sliced almonds, sprinkled with cinnamon and 1 teaspoon of vanilla extract; unsweetened green tea with lemon; a large glass of water

SNACK: 1 sliced apple with 2 tablespoons of peanut or nut butter**

LUNCH: Up to 6 ounces of grilled chicken over mixed greens, with sautéed mushrooms and Sugar Detox Vinaigrette*; a large glass of water

SNACK: Avocado with lemon and sliced red peppers, unsweetened green tea

DINNER: Green salad with 10 Mary's Gone Crackers, grilled shrimp with string beans, 1 (5-ounce) glass of red wine

SWEET SUCCESS
Rachel

"After I had my second baby, I was unable to get motivated to lose weight (although I loved to complain about it!). I ate, basically, like a fifteen-year-old boy, minus the fast food but with an addiction to Diet Coke and anything artificially sweetened—frozen yogurt, lots of Splenda in coffee, "diet" desserts and muffins, and so on. When I finally decided that I needed to lose weight, I tried the Sugar Detox. At first, I didn't think of it as a possible lifestyle change for me. No Diet Coke! No Splenda! No pizza! Not even fruit at first! . . . I thought that I would fall apart. The first three days were hard. I even got a headache from withdrawal from the Diet Coke. But something amazing happened: I lost 6 pounds in three days! After the first week, I felt much less bloated. After two weeks, I had lost 10 pounds. In three weeks, I went from wearing only maternity pants to wearing regular clothes. After four weeks, I had lost a total of 12.5 pounds and had totally changed the way that I eat. I have not felt hungry on this diet once. I don't always even eat all of the snacks. It's definitely hard—I would love more sweets and carbs, but that is what got me here in the first place! But I am totally satisfied and have been finding ways to incorporate some of my "treat" foods into the diet. I really cared about losing weight as my first priority—but perhaps the happiest surprise is that I really *feel* much better and healthier. I feel less sluggish throughout the day. My friends and family have noticed a huge difference, too. I owe all of my changes to the Sugar Detox plan."

WEEK 2 Add Some Fruit and an Extra Serving of Dairy

You're doing great, getting to Week 2 of the plan! By now, you've handled ten days of strict eating; during Week 2, you're going to start to loosen up a bit. Adding a portion of fruit for natural sugar (plus major skin benefits) will satisfy your sweet tooth. You might even be surprised just how sweet fruit actually tastes, now that your taste buds are sensitive to sugar! Oh, and enjoy some air-popped popcorn as a high-fiber snack—try sprinkling with some herbs if you miss traditional flavorings.

Week 2 Approved Foods
- 2 cups of unsweetened coffee per day max, plus 2 tablespoons 2% milk if desired
- Unsweetened green and/or herbal tea, in unlimited amounts
- Minimum 64 ounces of water (sodium-free sparkling water or club soda is okay)
- Protein: minimum 3 servings of lean red meat, pork, chicken, turkey, fish, shellfish, eggs, tofu, or legumes (see box on page 94 for vegetarian/vegan options; see serving sizes for protein on page 7)
- Dairy: 2 servings max of approved dairy (see page 96), plus an optional splash in coffee
- Vegetables: to the veggies approved for the 3-Day Sugar Fix and Week 1 (see pages 7 and 96), you may now add:
  - Carrots (cooked)
  - Jicama
  - Onions (cooked)
  - Peas (raw or cooked)

- Starchy vegetables: yam (1 small or ½ cup cubed) or summer squash (½ cup)
- Fruit: 1 medium-size apple; lemon or lime, for drinks or cooking; plus the following (serving size in parentheses):
  - Blackberries (½ cup)
  - Blueberries (½ cup)
  - Cantaloupe (½ cup)
  - Grapefruit (½ grapefruit)
  - Raspberries (½ cup)
  - Strawberries (½ cup)

- Nuts: a 1-ounce serving of nuts (see page 7) may be eaten up to twice daily as an additional snack.

- Seeds: a 1-ounce serving of sunflower or pumpkin seeds may be eaten up to twice daily as an additional snack.
- Popcorn: air-popped popcorn (1 cup) may be eaten daily as an additional snack.
- Fat: minimum 3 servings (from oils, olives, avocados, nuts, or seeds)
- Starch: 1 serving of approved-brand high-fiber crackers (2 crackers unless otherwise noted as a serving on the product label; (see approved-brands list, page 233)
- Alcohol: red wine only. 1 glass (5 fluid ounces) 3 times per week max
- Condiments and cooking oil: vinegar, olive oil, mustard, sesame oil, soy sauce

Cooking Techniques
- Sauté
- Steam
- Stir-fry
- Boil
- Poach

Remember to use only the oils on the approved list!

Week 2 Sample Daily Menu
See Chapter 13 or Recipe Index (page 257) for asterisked (*) recipes; if double-asterisked (**), see Appendix B for approved brands.

BREAKFAST: 3-egg omelet made with mozzarella cheese, mushrooms, and onions; 2 high-fiber crackers**; unsweetened coffee with a splash of 2% or whole milk; a large glass of water with lemon

SNACK: ½ cup of blueberries and 1 ounce of almonds, a large glass of water

LUNCH: Lentils with Sugar Detox Vinaigrette* over sautéed spinach, unsweetened mint green tea, a large glass of water

SNACK: Cottage cheese with apple slices, a large glass of water with lime

Alison arrived at the B Nutritious office with a typical patient story. She was overworked, over-tired, overbooked, and overweight. A high-profile

thirty-eight-year-old attorney, she kept long hours and many of her meals were with clients at restaurants or delivery to her office desk. For a 5-foot-7 woman, her weight was hovering at around 165 pounds and she felt awful. Formerly a soccer player in college, she had never worried about her weight until the last five years of long work hours had prevented her from any type of exercise. Alison was constantly taking over the counter anti-inflammatory pills for her headaches and joint pains and was using a steroid cream for the dry, patchy skin that would flare on her face and arms. Brooke assessed Alison and real-ized immediately that she was consuming huge amounts of sugar reg-ularly. Alison used diet soda to help her get through the day and was eating 100-calorie snack packs all day long. Brooke started Alison on the Sugar Detox, eliminating her beloved diet soft drinks, snack packs, and all other sugars. Within one week, Alison had stopped taking over-the-counter medicine for her headaches. Although her withdrawal symptoms were strong and she was fatigued and irritable the first three days, she stuck with it and was happy with the progression of her results. By the end of thirty-one days, Alison had lost just over 12 pounds. What was most remarkable were her energy level and her skin. She was now glowing and was no longer using steroids to help with her itchy, dry skin flare-ups. In fact, she hadn't had a flare-up since she started the diet. Alison remarked how much better her skin looked and how even her dark under-eye circles had diminished. She hadn't felt this well since college.

DINNER: Steamed artichoke with lemon-garlic vinaigrette, chicken and broccoli stir-fry, unsweetened cinnamon tea, a large glass of water with lemon

WEEK 3 Hello, Grains

By Week 3, it's time to reintroduce some healthy grains to your diet. We've found that our clients are sometimes apprehensive about doing this, nervous that the weight will come back on. Don't worry; we're adding healthy-portion-size, super-high-fiber grains that will help keep your blood sugar under control—and keep you satisfied!

And did we also mention that we're adding some chocolate?

Week 3 Approved Foods

- 2 cups of unsweetened coffee per day max, with only 2 tablespoons of 2% or whole milk if desired
- Unsweetened green and/or herbal tea, in unlimited amounts
- Minimum 64 ounces of water (sodium-free sparkling water or club soda is okay)
- Protein: minimum 3 servings of lean red meat, pork, chicken, turkey, fish, shellfish, eggs, tofu, or legumes (see box on page 94 for vegetarian/vegan options; see serving sizes for protein on page 7)
- Dairy: 2 servings max of approved dairy (see page 96), plus an optional splash in coffee
- Vegetable: the same veggies approved for the 3-Day Sugar Fix and Weeks 1 and 2 (see pages 7, 96, and 99)
- Starchy Vegetable: the same as in Week 2 (see page 99).
- Fruit: in addition to fruit from Week 2, 1 medium-size apple; lemon or lime, for drinks or cooking; plus one serving of the following (see, we told you it gets better!):
  - Cherries (½ cup, or 10 cherries)
  - Clementine (2 small clementines)
  - Grapes (½ cup)
  - Nectarine (1 nectarine)
  - Orange (1 medium-size orange)
  - Peach (1 peach)

- Nuts: a 1-ounce serving of nuts (see page 7) may be eaten up to twice daily as an additional snack.

- Seeds: a 1-ounce serving of sunflower or pumpkin seeds may be eaten up to twice daily as an additional snack.
- Popcorn: air-popped popcorn (1 cup) may be eaten daily as an additional snack.
- Fat: minimum 3 servings (from oils, olives, avocados, nuts, or seeds)
- Starch: 1 serving of approved-brand high-fiber crackers (2 crackers unless otherwise noted as a serving on the product label; (see approved-brands list, page 233), plus 1 serving of the following (check the product label for what constitutes a serving size):
  - Barley, ¼ cup uncooked, ½ cup cooked
  - Buckwheat, ¼ cup uncooked, ½ cup cooked, 2 oz soba noodles
  - Oatmeal (unsweetened; steel cut or rolled old-fashioned only, not instant), ¼ cup uncooked, ½ cup cooked
  - Protein-enriched pasta (see approved-brands list, page 237), 2 oz uncooked
  - Quinoa, ¼ cup uncooked, ½ cup cooked
  - Whole wheat pasta (see approved-brands list, page 237), 2 oz uncooked

- Alcohol: 1 glass (5 fluid ounces) of red wine only, four times per week max
- Dessert: dark chocolate (at least 65% cacao), 1 ounce per day
- Condiments and cooking oil: red wine vinegar, balsamic vinegar, or apple cider vinegar; and olive oil, coconut oil, or butter for cooking

Cooking Techniques
- Sauté
- Stir-fry
- Poach
- Steam
- Boil

Remember to use only the oils on the approved list!

Week 3 Sample Daily Menu
See Chapter 13 or Recipe Index (page 257) for asterisked (*) recipes; if double-asterisked (**), see Appendix B for approved brands.

BREAKFAST: ½ cup of cooked oatmeal, with 1 tablespoon of almond butter mixed in plus ½ cup of blueberries and 2 tablespoons of flaxseeds on top; unsweetened green tea; a large glass of water with lime

SNACK: 1 apple with string cheese, a large glass of sparkling water

LUNCH: tuna and string bean salad with Sugar Detox Vinaigrette* and 2 high-fiber crackers**, a large glass of water with lemon

SNACK: guacamole and carrots, unsweetened mint tea

DINNER: a large warm chicken salad: poached chicken on top of mixed greens and goat cheese, with mustard dressing; 2 large Dark Chocolate–Covered Strawberries*

SWEET SUCCESS
Phil

"I was an athlete with an attention-getting physique well through my thirties. Over the past fifteen years I've gained over 50 pounds. My blood pressure was high because of it, and I was feeling out of control. My energy was down, almost as low as my self-esteem. It's been years since I have gone swimming or to the beach—I was too embarrassed to let anyone see how overweight I was. I heard about the Sugar Detox on a Sunday, and started it on the next day. I lost 23 pounds in the first thirty-one days! The plan is surprisingly easy to follow—it has very clear and simple guidelines. It is especially practical for someone with a job as demanding and stressful as mine—I need a plan with easy rules. Although the first three weeks are fairly strict, the plan is presented in a way that helps you look beyond the initial phases. And the plan is based both on excellent nutrition and the fail-proof principle of eliminating natural and artificial sugars from my diet. Because the plan helps you add back in some treat foods, it is easy to stay motivated. Dark chocolate has never tasted so good! Thank you, Sugar Detox. For the first time in years, I feel like I am getting control back over myself. My energy level has improved, and so has my mood."

WEEK 4 Keep the Momentum

This is the home stretch! Week 4 is a step away from how to continue living on the Sugar Detox. You'll still be losing weight this week, but you'll certainly be satisfied with all the extras you now get to eat. More starches and more fruit!

Week 4 Approved Foods

- 2 cups of unsweetened coffee per day max, with only 2 table-spoons of 2% or whole milk if desired
- Unsweetened green and/or herbal tea, in unlimited amounts
- Minimum 64 ounces of water (sodium-free sparkling water or club soda is okay)
- Protein: minimum 3 servings of lean red meat, pork, chicken, turkey, fish, shellfish, eggs, tofu, or legumes (see box on page 94 for vegetarian/vegan options; see serving sizes for protein on page 7)
- Dairy: 2 servings max of approved dairy (see page 96), plus an optional splash in coffee
- Vegetable: the same veggies approved for the 3-Day Sugar Fix and Weeks 1 and 2 (see pages 7, 96, and 99)
- Starchy Vegetable: the same as in Weeks 2 and 3 (see page 99)
- Fruit: 1 medium-size apple; lemon or lime, for drinks or cooking plus one and a half servings of the approved fruits from Weeks 2 and 3 (see page 102)
- Nuts: a 1-ounce serving of nuts (see page 7) may be eaten twice daily as an additional snack.
- Seeds: a 1-ounce serving of sunflower or pumpkin seeds may be eaten twice daily as an additional snack.
- Popcorn: air-popped popcorn (1 cup) may be eaten daily as an additional snack.
- Fat: minimum 3 servings (from oils, olives, avocados, nuts, or seeds)
- Starch: 2 servings per day of starches added in Weeks 3 and 4 (see page 103), plus 1 serving of approved-brand high-fiber crackers

(2 crackers unless otherwise noted as a serving on the product label; (see approved-brands list, page 233), plus 1 serving of the following (check the product label for what constitutes a serving size):

○ Breads (see approved-brands list, page 233)
○ Cereals (see approved-brands list, page 234)
○ Brown rice

- Alcohol: 1 glass (5 fluid ounces) of red wine only, five glasses max per week
- Dessert: dark chocolate (at least 65% cacao), 1 ounce per day
- Condiments and cooking oil: red wine vinegar, balsamic vinegar, or apple cider vinegar; and olive oil, coconut oil, or butter for cooking

Cooking Techniques
- Sauté
- Steam
- Stir-fry
- Boil
- Poach

Remember to use only the oils on the approved list!

Week 4 Sample Daily Menu
See Chapter 13 or Recipe Index (page 257) for asterisked (*) recipes; if double-asterisked (**), see Appendix B for approved brands.

BREAKFAST: open BTA sandwich: 1 slice multigrain bread with 2 slices turkey bacon, a slice of tomato, and ¼ avocado; ½ grapefruit; unsweetened green tea with lemon; a large glass of water

SNACK: ½ cup part-skim ricotta cheese with sliced apple, sprinkled with cinnamon; a large glass of water with lime

LUNCH: 3-bean chili with high-fiber crackers**, unsweetened ginger-cinnamon tea, a large glass of water

SNACK: 1 ounce roasted pumpkin seeds, 1 orange, unsweetened green tea, a large glass of water

DINNER: Bibb leaf salad with feta cheese, grapes, and celery, with Sugar Detox Vinaigrette*; arctic char with olives, capers, and lemon, 1 ounce of dark chocolate (65% cacao minimum); a large glass of water

Now that you've kicked your sugar habit, you'll notice that you have more energy, feel less bloated . . . and your skin glows! Read on for more information about how you can maximize those efforts to rejuvenate your skin even more. You'll also find more tips for long-term Sugar Detox maintenance, as well as a companion exercise plan.

9

Your Dermal Detox

If you follow our Sugar Detox plan, you'll notice changes in both the way you feel and look. As you know by now, what you put in your body really shows up in your skin. Our skin-care regimen is designed to work in tandem with the four-week diet program so you truly can reap its benefits inside and out.

Our simple daily regimen should be started on the first day of Week 1; it will keep your skin healthy and maintain a youthful glow. It's fairly simple to make our plan a part of your daily life—just two steps in the morning and two steps at night—to ensure your skin is protected from damaging free radicals and protein glycation, and to repair any damage that has already been done. The morning regimen is designed to protect your skin, whereas the evening regimen will repair while you sleep.

Here's a basic chart that outlines the Sugar Detox daily skin regimen that will help you look as great on the outside as you feel on the inside. If you haven't yet gotten started, you might want to review our recommended skin-care shopping list on page 241.

Step 1: Cleansing Morning and Evening with Gentle Exfoliation

The first step every morning and evening is cleansing. The skin's upper layer (epidermis) is composed of living and dead cells. As the epidermal cells grow and divide, older cells are pushed up to the surface of the skin, where they eventually die and flake off. This dead cell layer that lies on

TABLE 9.1 Daily Skin-care Regimen

	SKIN TYPE		
	Sensitive skin	Normal to Dry	Oily or acne prone
STEP 1: AM/PM Equipment and cleaners	Soft washcloth with gentle cleanser. Look for "sensitive skin" on the label.	Soft washcloth with a cleanser that contains glycolic acid, maltobionic or gluconolactone. OR Once or twice weekly exfoliation with cleansing brush, and a bland cleanser (without AHAs or BHAs).	Soft washcloth with a cleanser that contains glycolic acid or salicylic acid. Astringent or toner optional. OR Once or twice weekly exfoliation with cleansing brush, bland cleanser OR do a weekly or biweekly granular scrub.
STEP 2a: AM Morning cosmeceutical to protect against glycation and free radical damage	Serum or cream with antioxidants	Serum or cream antioxidants	Serum with antioxidants
STEP 2b: AM Sun protection	Zinc oxide and/or titanium dioxide. Look for products labeled chemical free or sensitive skin.	Zinc oxide and/or, titanium dioxide, or traditional organic sunscreens	Light traditional organic sunscreen (oil-free lotion or gel based)
STEP 2c: PM Evening cosmeceutical for skin repair	Moisturizer with repairing ingredients; avoid retinol/retinoic acid, glycolic/lactic, salicylic acid	Moisturizer with repairing ingredients, including retinol/retinoic acid cream	Moisturizer with repairing ingredients, including retinol/retinoic acid cream or gel

the surface of the skin is called the stratum corneum, or keratin layer. As we age, this process of growing, dividing, and flaking off slows down. Dead cells that remain on the surface leave skin looking uneven, dry, and patchy. These cells also reflect light, causing the skin to look dull, and clogging pores, exacerbating breakouts.

It is essential to cleanse facial skin to remove dirt, pollution, surface oils, and makeup. As a dermatologist, Dr. Farris can tell you that it is downright shocking how many patients will admit that they do not regularly cleanse their face. This is especially true of women, who often flop into bed at night without even washing off their makeup. Okay, we know you're tired, but this is not an option! All that dirt and grime builds up over time, putting added and unnecessary stress on the skin. And there's a flip side to this: Some women—most of whom have oily and acne-prone skin—wash too much, trying to remove their blemishes with aggressive scrubs. Believe us, it doesn't work! Dr. Farris always tells them, "If you could wash pimples away, dermatologists would be out of business."

The most basic skin care regimen should include twice-daily cleansing. Gentle daily exfoliation helps remove dead skin cells, leaving skin looking smoother and more radiant. Exfoliation also helps enhance the penetration of therapeutic skin-care products, making it a win-win in our book. The secret here is *gentle* exfoliation. Cleansing should be the mildest step in your skin care routine, as it is simply used to prepare the skin for your treatment regimen. Aggressive exfoliation can actually damage the skin barrier, leaving skin dry and irritated. If you have supersensitive skin or suffer from rosacea or any other facial dermatitis, even gentle exfoliation may cause irritation and exacerbate redness. In this case, we suggest you forgo the exfoliation and cleanse with a mild sensitive skin cleanser applied to the face with a soft cloth or fingertips.

There are two kinds of exfoliation: mechanical and chemical. Mechanical exfoliation physically removes dead skin cells, whereas chemical exfoliation dissolves them. In general, mechanical exfoliation is too aggressive for daily use, so we suggest you use this only once or twice weekly. Chemical exfoliation is milder and more appropriate for daily use.

Chemical Exfoliation

Chemical exfoliation can be achieved by using cleansers that contain one of the following hydroxy acids: glycolic acid, salicylic acid, or gluconolactone. When applied to the skin, these gently dissolve the glue that holds dead skin cells together, promoting a gentle chemical exfoliation. Salicylic acid, a form of beta hydroxy acid (BHA), is best for oily and acne-prone skin. Glycolic acid is an alpha hydroxy acid (AHA); cleansers with this ingredient are used extensively by dermatologists as part of an anti-aging regimen. But for those with sensitive skin, these ingredients can cause irritation. On the other hand, gluconolactone, a polyhydroxy acid, is one of the mildest chemical exfoliators. Cleansers that contain gluconolactone can be used on all skin types, including sensitive skin. The newest hydroxy acids, the bionic acids, include maltobionic and lactobionic acid and are gentle and effective chemical exfoliators. See our list of recommended cleansers (Appendix C).

Mechanical Exfoliation

Mechanical exfoliation should be used once or twice a week. For mechanical exfoliation, we suggest you use a soft cleansing brush, or a cleansing cloth or mitt specially intended for the face. Most of the major cosmetic companies now market these types of cleansing aids. They are inexpensive, safe, and effective. Handheld electric cleansing brushes are creating quite a buzz and can be found in drugstores and department stores. There are basically two types to choose from. Rotary-type brushes go around in a circular motion, while oscillating brushes move back and forth. So what's the difference? Well cost, for one thing. The oscillating brushes are more expensive, but they do have more bells and whistles and are viewed as gentler on the skin. Some oscillating brushes can be fitted with a variety of brush heads, including options for those with sensitive and acne-prone skin, making them a winner in our book. Studies have been conducted on both rotary and oscillating cleansing brushes and show that they remove makeup effectively and reduce surface oils, all while cleansing the skin. It's important when using an electric cleansing brush not to apply too much pressure to the skin, as this can cause irritation. Also, cleansing brushes of any kind should not be used on skin that is infected or has any type of open wounds. Cleansing brushes should be used with your favorite gentle cleanser. These brushes have really revolutionized the way we care for our faces and are now recommended by dermatologists in the know, to be used as part of your skin care regimen. And, trust us, once you have one, you won't remember how you lived without it. These make exfoliation an enjoyable spa-like experience, leaving skin smooth without irritation. It's important to say that mechanical exfoliation is not for all skin types; see Table 9.1 for more specific instructions based on your skin type.

If you are acne prone, or your skin is very oily, or you have clogged pores, you may benefit from an alternative type of mechanical exfoliation using a granular cleanser once a week. Granular cleansers have a slightly gritty feel to them, thanks to their tiny beads that exfoliate the skin. If you want to maximize the benefits of a granular scrub, apply it when you are in a hot shower and your pores are open. Gently massage the cleanser into your skin with your fingertips for two to three minutes before rinsing.

We've seen women who've tried using chemical and mechanical exfoliation together. We strongly discourage this as it can lead to excessively dry and irritated skin. For this reason, we recommend you either use a soft washcloth and one of the hydroxy acid cleansers appropriate for your skin type mentioned above, or select a bland cleanser (without AHAs or BHAs) to use daily and with your cleansing brush once or twice a week. Also, if you are using a vitamin A cream at night, remember this makes skin more fragile; so skip your nightly application for a day or two prior to mechanical exfoliation.

Toners and Astringents May Be Unnecessary

What about toners and astringents? Toners and astringents were originally designed to remove soap residue from the skin. They are leave-on liquids that are applied to the face with a cotton ball after cleansing.

While many women remain devoted to this second step of the cleansing regimen, in reality these products are obsolete. Most modern cleansing products leave virtually no soap residue, thus eliminating the need for toners and astringents. Of course, there is always an exception to every rule. If you have oily skin and are acne prone, this second step may be of value in that it removes residual surface oils, leaving skin feeling squeaky clean.

Step 2a Morning: Prevent Glycation and Oxidative Damage

The first product that should be put on your skin after cleansing in the morning is an antioxidant. Antioxidants can be applied as serums or creams, and may even be included in some of the newer sunscreen products. These antioxidant products will serve to protect your skin from free radical damage and glycation. Serums are a favorite of ours, as they are light, don't clog pores, and can be used to deliver a concentrate of antioxidants to the skin. Serums can also be applied under moisturizer, makeup, or sunscreen, making them a perfect way to start protecting your skin in the morning. Many products are supercharged with a combination of antioxidants that work synergistically. Reasonably priced antioxidants can be found in drugstores, cosmetic stores, day spas, and dermatologist offices. Air and light can degrade antioxidants, so look for products in dark or opaque bottles with a pump that can keep air out. We recommend you choose an antioxidant product that contains at least one of our all-star glycation inhibitors, or even better, one that contains several of them: rosemary extract, thyme extract, resveratrol, green or black tea extract, curcumin, phloretin, quercetin, pomegranate extract, blueberry extract, seaweed extract, L-carnosine, and alpha lipoic acid. All of these will be discussed later in this chapter (see pages 124–131).

Step 2b Morning: Sun Protection

Remember, antioxidants are not meant to be a substitute for sunscreen but used in addition to sunscreen; the latter actually absorb or block rays as they enter the skin, so they provide a totally different type of protection than an antioxidant product does. When choosing a sunscreen, make sure you are using one with a sun-protection factor (SPF) of no less than 30, and choose one that is even higher if you are planning a day of outdoor activities. It is also essential that your sunscreen be labeled "broad spectrum" and contain ingredients that block both ultraviolet A (UVA) and ultraviolet B (UVB) rays. Sunscreens are classified based on how they protect the skin. Organic sunscreens, also called chemical sunscreens, use a combination of chemicals to absorb ultraviolet light while inorganic sunscreens—physical blockers—use particles to reflect and scatter ultraviolet light. Physical sunscreens that offer micronized forms of zinc or titanium dioxide are an excellent choice, as these particles can block both UVA and UVB rays. Tinted varieties are also available and are great for those with darker skin tones. There are many cosmetically elegant sunscreens to choose from and some of the best can be purchased at the drugstore without breaking the bank.

> *Sweet **Talk***
> Dr. F says:
>
> *"Those brown spots that women hate on the back of their hands are not age spots, they are sun spots."*

All-Star Sunscreen Ingredients

UVA protection: avobenzone (Parsol 1789) or a stabilized form called Helioplex, ecamsule (Mexoryl™ SX)

UVB protection: homosalate, octyl salicylate, octocrylene, octyl methoxycinnamate, cinoxate, oxybenzone, dioxybenzone, sulisobenzone, menthyl anthranilate

UVA and UVB protection: titanium dioxide, zinc oxide

Step 2c Evening: Repair by Using Moisturizers with a Kick

This part of our evening regimen will give new meaning to the term *beauty sleep*. After cleansing we recommend using a moisturizer that will help repair and rehydrate your skin. Why is moisturizing so important? As it turns out, moisturizers have real benefits when it comes to skin health and beauty. Dry skin is patchy, dull, and looks more wrinkled. Studies have shown that by applying nothing more than a bland moisturizer, you can temporarily improve skin wrinkling as much as 10 to 15 percent. This is because moisturizers keep water in the skin, plumping it and making wrinkles less noticeable. Moisturizers also help protect the skin barrier function, preventing chaffing, irritation, and infection. So moisturizing is an essential step in our regimen for keeping skin healthy and beautiful. The following is a guide to choosing moisturizers; once you find one that suits you, it should be applied nightly after your evening cleanse.

Moisturizing Basics

We know there are tons of products out there, so first we're going to demystify moisturizers. Dr. Farris often gets asked, do more expensive moisturizers work better? The answer is absolutely not, because all moisturizers are basically formulated the same. The main difference in pricing comes from the bells and whistles, such as fancy packaging and celebrity endorsements. All moisturizers contain three main components: occlusives, humectants, and emollients, which are combined with water, thickeners, preservatives, and fragrance. Although many seek out moisturizers that are preservative- and fragrance-free, this may go against conventional wisdom. The right preservatives are necessary to enhance shelf life and prevent contamination. If you are a less-is-more kind of girl, fragrance-free might suit your fancy, but in general, fragrance is fine as long as you are not allergic to it. True fragrance allergy is tricky, as products that are unscented may still actually contain fragrance to mask the odor of chemicals in the formulation. If you suspect you have fragrance allergy, this can be confirmed by patch testing that can be performed by your dermatologist.

Occlusive ingredients are the oily substances in moisturizers that prevent water loss by forming barrier on the surface of the skin. They seal in water so that it is not lost to the environment, thus improving skin

So Many Products . . . Which to Choose?

Dr. Farris has been studying cosmeceutical skin-care products and their active ingredients for over twenty years. She serves as a consultant to major cosmetic companies and has lectured and published on the science behind these unique skin-care products. Cosmeceuticals are skin-care products that contain active benefit ingredients that provide real improvements in the appearance of skin. So in essence, the products we will discuss are a blend between cosmetics and pharmaceuticals, providing added benefits over those that are mere cosmetics. Most of the early cosmeceuticals contained only one active ingredient, such as vitamin C or retinol, but today most products offer a combination of unique ingredients that work synergistically, giving you more bang for the buck. When shopping for cosmeceuticals, some simple tips can help as you navigate through the vast number of products on the shelf and the Internet. Here are some tips that we hope will help you avoid cosmeceutical confusion and those all-too-common cosmetic counter conundrums:

- Higher prices don't necessarily mean a better or more effective product.
- Choose major consumer brands and avoid products from obscure sources.
- When reading the label, keep in mind that ingredients are listed in order of decreasing concentration—the most plentiful ingredient is listed first.
- Never forget that the salesperson behind a department store counter is employed by the cosmetic line, so take the advice with a grain of salt.
- If the claims on a product seem too good to be true, they probably are.

hydration. Some of the more commonly used ingredients include petrolatum, lanolin, mineral oil, beeswax, and the silicone derivatives dimethicone and cyclomethicone. If a product is labeled "oil-free," this generally means that it does not contain petrolatum, mineral, or vegetable oils. Alternatively, oil-free moisturizers will use one of the silicone derivatives, such as dimethicone, as an occlusive.

Humectants are compounds that, like tiny sponges, attract water from the dermis and lower epidermis to hydrate the upper epidermis and its outermost layer, the stratum corneum. When the humidity is over 70 percent, humectants can draw water from the environment, hydrating the skin from the outside in. Humectants must be used in combination with occlusive agents so that the water they attract into the stratum corneum will not evaporate into the environment. Glycerin, hyaluronic acid, sodium lactate, urea, and honey are some of the more commonly used humectant ingredients. Propylene glycol is a commonly used humectant with antibacterial properties. While this ingredient may cause skin irritation, it is less likely to cause true allergic reactions.

You know how smooth and silky your skin feels after you moisturize? Well, that's because of the third component of moisturizers: emollients. Emollients fill in the spaces between the dead skin cells, decreasing skin friction and leaving a smoother skin surface. Some of the more commonly used emollients include jojoba oil, sunflower seed oil, and palm oil. If you have been seeking out skin-care products that are alcohol-free, you might be surprised to know several alcohols serve as emollient moisturizers; examples include cetyl alcohol and stearyl alcohol. These alcohols are included in moisturizers because they leave skin feeling silky and smooth. If the alcohol content of your skin-care products matters to you, read the ingredients on the label carefully for such terms.

All moisturizers are formulated as emulsions, meaning they are a mixture of oil and water. Lotions have more water than oil, whereas creams have a higher oil content. Their greater oil content is why creams are thicker than lotions. Many people prefer lotions to creams in the summer but use creams when it's colder and drier. This makes sense, as cold and low humidity dehydrate the skin. More mature women often have drier skin and tend to prefer creams. If you are acne prone, stick to products labeled "oil-free." In the end, when you choose a moisturizer you have to consider your climate, the time of year, and any preexisting skin conditions you might have.

Moisturizers That Repair

Now that you are a pro at moisturizer basics, let's talk about some of the ingredients that can be used to enhance the benefits of moisturizers. Plenty of ingredients claim to turn back the hands of time, but many of these are nothing more than hope in a jar. To save you the time and money, we have done the homework for you. Our list includes ingredients that can truly improve the appearance of aging skin.

VITAMIN A GETS AN A

Vitamin A and its derivatives are among the most valued compounds in dermatology. Also called retinol, vitamin A has been used extensively for treating aging skin and is available in many over-the-counter moisturizers. Once inside the skin, retinol is converted to the active form of vitamin A called retinoic acid. Retinoic acid repairs skin by attaching to receptors that turn on and off certain cellular functions—specifically, turning on collagen production and turning off collagen breakdown. This increase in dermal collagen is why retinol does such a great job at softening fine lines and wrinkles. Cosmeceuticals containing retinol also lighten pigmentation, reduce the appearance of pores, and improve tone and texture. Look for products that contain retinol or its derivatives; it is generally agreed that retinol itself is the most effective form of vitamin A in over-the-counter products, followed by the derivatives retinaldehyde, retinyl proprionate, and retinyl palmitate, in that order.

The real deal, retinoic acid, is available only by prescription, under such trade names as Retina A, Renova, or Refissa. If you prefer generic products, this product will be labeled "tretinoin" (the *t* stands for "trans"). While the over-the counter derivatives discussed earlier are effective, they are far less potent than these prescription products. Studies have shown that retinoic acid creams rejuvenate skin by firming and smoothing. Retinoic acid also regulates cell turnover, shedding dead skin cells and leaving skin brighter and more radiant.

So here's the big question dermatologists so often get asked: Should I buy something over the counter or go to my doctor for a prescription? Dr. Farris usually recommends starting with an over-the-counter vitamin A product, especially if you have sensitive or mature skin. These OTC options are less potent yet still effective. They are also far less irritating. If your skin is oily or acne prone, though, you may be better served with prescription tretinoin. It is important to note that several other prescription forms of vitamin A, including tazarotene and adapalene, are used to treat aging skin. This is where your dermatologist can be helpful in guiding you with product selection. (Products containing prescription forms of vitamin A should not be used during pregnancy.)

VITAMIN B3 (NIACINAMIDE)

Niacinamide is one of the most valuable ingredients used in anti-aging cosmeceuticals and is great for all skin types, including sensitive skin. Niacinamide improves skin hydration by increasing important skin lipids such as ceramides, thus improving barrier function. Niacinamide also reduces oil production from oil glands and improves the appearance of pore size. Products containing niacinamide have been shown to soften fine lines and wrinkles, lighten mottled pigmentation and reduce sallowness. The icing on the cake is that this vitamin is a precursor to a potent antioxidant that inhibits protein glycation. We suggest you add this to your list of ingredients to look for since it can both repair and protect aging skin.

VITAMIN C: SUNSHINE VITAMIN IS GOOD FOR SKIN, TOO!

Topical vitamin C, applied in serums and creams, is a favorite of dermatologists because it does so many good things for your skin. Vitamin C is a potent skin antioxidant and anti-inflammatory. It turns on the enzymes that produce collagen, so it is essential to maintaining a healthy

---

Side Effects with Retinoic Acid and Retinol

It's important to understand that when you first starting using retinoic acid or even retinol, your skin may get pink and a little flaky. This common side effect, called retinoid dermatitis, usually lasts just a couple of weeks as the skin gets used to the product. Gentle exfoliation will help remove flaky skin and applying a rich hydrating cream several times a day will combat the dryness. We suggest you start vitamin A creams every other night for the first several weeks, to minimize retinoid dermatitis. While many believe that you are more sensitive to the sun when using a topical vitamin A cream, there is really very little scientific evidence to support this notion. We do suggest that you wear a daily sunscreen when using these products, to prevent further sun damage. Also, remember to stop using any type of vitamin A cream five to seven days prior to waxing or having any type of in-office skin-related procedure, including laser treatments and chemical peels.

---

supporting structure for your skin. Also, Vitamin C lightens pigmentation and improves skin tone, making it a great option for treating sun-damaged skin. Look for cosmeceutical products containing ascorbyl phosphate, ascorbyl-6-palmitate, ascorbyl tetraisopalmitate, or L-ascorbic acid. These ingredients will help improve fine lines and wrinkles and restore to your skin its youthful glow.

PEPTIDES—PROTEINS THAT PERK UP COLLAGEN

Collagen-boosting peptides are an interesting new category of over-the-counter cosmeceutical ingredients. The first peptides marketed were small fragments of collagen that were shown to enhance collagen production by fibroblasts (the dermal cells that make collagen). Cosmeceutical moisturizers containing these peptides were tested in human skin and found to improve fine lines and wrinkles with continued use.

These peptides are currently marketed under the trade names Matrixyl and Matrixyl 3000, and can be found in many popular over-the-counter cosmeceuticals. Both of these ingredients will enhance collagen production, helping to rejuvenate skin while you sleep. One of the advantages to peptide cosmeceuticals is that the ingredients are nonirritating, so they are well tolerated even if you have sensitive skin or cannot tolerate vitamin A creams.

HYDROXY ACIDS—MORE THAN JUST EXFOLIATION

We talked about hydroxy acids and their value as exfoliators in cleansers, but these ingredients can also be used in moisturizers that will improve the appearance of aging skin. While we still recommend products with glycolic and lactic acid, some newer-generation hydroxy acids are milder and more effective. These compounds, called bionic acids, are third-generation hydroxy acids that have unique moisturizing properties, in that they attract water to the skin. Bionic acids also act as antioxidants, but even more important, they rev up the synthesis of hyaluronic acid. Hyaluronic acid is the stuff that makes babies' cheeks chubby and it essential for keeping our skin chubby, too. Studies of bionic acids have shown them to be effective for softening fine lines and wrinkles and improving skin's appearance. The key ingredients you should look for are lactobionic acid and maltobionic acid.

N-ACETYLGLUCOSAMINE—PLUMP IT UP!

N-acetylglucosamine is a relative newcomer to cosmeceutical skin care. This molecule is a building block of hyaluronic acid and plumps skin from the inside out. Studies have shown that women using this novel ingredient had significant anti-aging benefits including improvement in fine lines and wrinkles, skin pigmentation and roughness. As an added benefit, N-acetylglucosamine has been shown to improve acne when compared to the market leader benzoyl peroxide. This skin-repairing ingredient gets a gold star in our book for being both effective and gentle enough for all skin types. Look for products with either N-acetylglucosamine or NeoGlucosamine.

Natural Skin Care from Land and Sea

As you already know, we value natural ingredients. The Sugar Detox diet places a heavy emphasis on deriving health benefits from natural food sources. So it should come as no surprise that when it comes to topical skin care, we prefer naturals as well. We believe that naturals are among the most effective skin-care ingredients, giving your skin powerful yet gentle anti-aging solutions.

Many of the natural ingredients we will be talking about are what we call multitaskers, meaning they function in more than one way. These multifunctional ingredients pack a powerful punch that can improve skin's appearance, fight the visible signs of aging, and stop skin glycation. This is why we are giving them a top spot on our list of all-star ingredients. With our focus on naturals, it is important to say that we are not against synthetic ingredients, as there are many excellent synthetic ingredients that can work wonders on the skin.

That said, plants, or botanicals, are one of the most valuable natural resources for skin-care ingredients. Plants can be cultivated, grown, and harvested to ensure that they are rich in vitamins, emollients, and antioxidants. To be used in a skin-care product, plants must be processed into extracts, which usually involves pressing or grinding the plant. Extracts must be prepared carefully to make sure that the ingredients remain active, so that the product you're using actually has more of a purpose than just smelling great.

As we discussed earlier, oxidative stress causes skin aging by ramping up skin inflammation, glycation, and collagen breakdown. The use of topical antioxidants to neutralize free radicals and prevent oxidative damage is well supported by scientific studies. Plants, like humans, are armed with an antioxidant defense system. Plants grow in sunlight and use antioxidants to protect themselves from sun-induced damaging free radicals. Polyphenols, as discussed in Chapter 5, are unique antioxidants that are found in plants. These colorful antioxidant compounds are found in plant extracts and can be formulated for use in skin-care products. Cosmetic chemists favor plant-based antioxidants because they can be obtained from almost any part of a plant, including the bark, stems, leaves, seeds, and flowers.

Dermatologists now routinely recommend topical antioxidants to protect skin from free radicals and glycation. Studies have shown that topical antioxidants can prevent sunburn, and stave off the signs of premature skin aging. Cosmeceuticals with antioxidants can be used to prevent skin inflammation, so they can also be helpful in treating such skin conditions as rosacea and acne.

What follows are some of the botanical sources of powerful natural extracts that can be used to fight glycation and skin aging.

All-Star Botanical Glycation Inhibitors

HERBS AND SPICES

Herbs and spices have been used for centuries as alternative medications. They have been used to control weight, lower blood sugar levels, reduce inflammation, and treat arthritis and joint pain, as well as make hair and skin healthier. They can also provide health benefits such as reducing the likelihood of getting high blood pressure, cataracts, and even cancer. The miraculous properties of herbs and spices are due primarily to their antioxidants and healing properties.

Herbs and spices are powerful glycation inhibitors. In a study comparing twenty-four herbal and spice extracts, spices were found to be among the most potent for inhibiting glycation, although many commonly used herbs were also effective. We have included many of these in our diet plan and recipes, as they add flavor and can help reduce glycation from the inside out, for a more youthful appearance.

Rosemary (*Rosmarinus officinalis*). Rosemary is a common household herb known for its unique fragrance and flavor. Rosemary extract, which is made from the tiny leaves of the rosemary bush, has potent antioxidant and antibacterial activity and inhibits metalloproteinase enzymes, which break down collagen. Rosemary leaf extract protects skin from free radical damage and prevents oxidative stress. Laboratory studies have confirmed the ability of rosemary extract to inhibit collagen glycation, making it useful for preventing skin aging.

Thyme (*Thymus vulgaris*). This spice is great on turkey, but its healing powers might surprise you. Thyme contains a variety of polyphenols called flavonoids. Thyme extract acts as an anti-inflammatory, and a recent study pending publication suggests that thyme can kill bacteria, too. The scientists conducting this research compared thyme extract to the commonly used acne medication benzoyl peroxide for killing bacteria. Much to their surprise, the thyme extract outperformed benzoyl peroxide, making it a potential alternative for treating acne. Thyme extract is also a potent glycation inhibitor, so when we say thyme is good for your skin, you can see we are not just talking turkey.

Turmeric (*Curcuma longa*). Turmeric is a medicinal herb that has long been used in Chinese medicine. The roots are ground into a powder, yielding the spice that is used as flavoring for foods such as curry. Turmeric contains the active ingredient curcumin, the polyphenolic antioxidant that gives it its distinctive yellow color. Curcumin promotes wound healing, has natural antibacterial activity, and acts as an anti-inflammatory agent. As a polyphenol, curcumin is one of the most potent antioxidants for preventing glycation. In some recent preliminary studies curcumin was compounded in a gel base and applied to the skin. This herbal gel was shown to prevent and decrease scar tissue formation following surgery, as well as to improve sun damage, including reducing the appearance of wrinkles. Improvement in sun-damaged skin occurred after using the product for three to six months. The greatest improvement was seen in those with more severe sun damage. With all of these exciting studies, topical curcumin holds promise as a cosmeceutical agent for treating aging skin.

TEA (CAMELLIA SINENSIS)

Green Tea. Green tea has been used extensively for medicinal purposes for centuries and is an all-star food on the Sugar Detox list. Green tea

Quercetin—Your Antiglycation Superhero

Quercetin is one of the most plentiful flavonols in our diet, found in red apples as well as green and black tea, capers, red onions, red grapes, and some berries. Like other flavonoids, quercetin has broad biologic activity, including anti-inflammatory activity and prevention of cancer. Quercetin has been shown to inhibit glycation of DNA in experimental models. Cosmeceuticals containing quercetin can be used to treat skin aging, sun damage, and inflammatory skin conditions such as acne.

polyphenols (GTPs) are among the most potent antioxidants and have been shown to have antiglycation properties. Studies have confirmed that ingestion of green tea extract effectively blocks collagen cross-linking and inhibits AGE accumulation associated with aging. Green tea can also be prepared as an extract for use in cosmeceutical skin care. Topical green tea extract protects against UV-induced inflammation and oxidative stress, making it a powerful, topical skin care agent. Using skin-care products containing GTPs is an excellent way to inhibit collagen glycation and protect skin from damaging UV rays.

White and Black Tea. Although green tea contains the most potent antioxidants, white tea is a close second. Black tea is less potent than green or white, but still contains enough antioxidants to make it a valuable cosmeceutical ingredient. You will find extracts of white and black teas in serums, lotions, and masks designed to protect the skin from the effects of free radicals.

FRUITS AND VEGETABLES

Apples. Apples are known to have numerous health benefits, including prevention of cancer, heart disease, and diabetes. Phloretin is a flavonoid antioxidant found exclusively in apples and apple products. Phloretin and its sister compound phloridzin have both been found to have antidiabetic effects. They inhibit intestinal absorption of glucose and have been shown to prevent AGE formation. Cosmeceuticals with phloretin can be used to inhibit oxidative stress and protect collagen from glycation.

Blueberries. Blueberry extract contains antioxidant flavonoids and has been shown to inhibit glycation. Studies have evaluated a cosmeceutical product containing blueberry extract and other anti-aging ingredients. The product was tested on diabetic women who had moderate to severe sun damage. After twelve weeks of applying the test product two times a day, investigators found significant improvement in skin hydration, skin thickness, fine lines, firmness, radiance, crepiness, and overall appearance. It's no surprise that blueberry extract is now gaining popularity among dermatologists as an antioxidant and anti-aging ingredient.

Grapes. As we've already discussed, red grapes are an excellent source of resveratrol. Interest in resveratrol started back in the early 1990s, when it was first noted that the French had a very low incidence of heart disease—yet the French diet was notably high in fats. *The French paradox*, as it was dubbed, was later explained by the fact that the French also consumed lots of red wine, which is full of resveratrol. More recent studies have shown that resveratrol isn't the only antioxidant in red wine; it also contains other polyphenols, which have been shown to have protective effects on blood vessels, keeping them healthy and preventing heart disease. But you don't need to drink wine to reap the benefits of red grapes. Resveratrol-containing cosmeceuticals are widely available and are a great way to give your skin extra antioxidant protection and prevent glycation.

Pomegranate (*Punica granatum*). Pomegranate is an ancient fruit known for its skin rejuvenating benefits. Pomegranate seed oil promotes regeneration of the upper layer of the skin while extracts of pomegranate peel regenerate the lower layer, turning on collagen production and inhibiting collagen-digesting enzymes. Extract of the rind of pomegranate inhibits glycation, turns off pigment production and acts as an antioxidant. The diverse beauty benefits of this fruit have made it a favorite for use in anti-aging cosmeceuticals.

Sea-Derived Cosmeceuticals

There is growing interest in our oceans as a resource for anti-aging compounds. To date, over six thousand biologically active molecules have
been harvested from sea life. Many of these molecules possess medicinal powers. They have been used to control high blood pressure, treat
liver disease, act as antibiotics, and function as blood thinners. The use
of sea life for treating aging skin is an evolving field in dermatology and
represents a new frontier in cosmeceuticals. Much like plants found on
land, plants living under the sea are a rich source of antioxidants. These
compounds create the beautiful colors that exist on coral reefs and undersea landscapes. Sea animals and birds that graze the ocean floor, eating plants and algae, ingest these antioxidants, using them as nutrients.
Once ingested, these compounds impart their hues to the creatures that
eat them, turning crustaceans such as lobsters red and making flamin-
gos brightly colored. The following are some all-star anti-aging compounds from the sea.

SEAWEED

Algae, or seaweed, are one of the most plentiful resources in nature.
Algae can be found in fresh and saltwater and in both unicellular and
multicellular forms. Often confused with plants, seaweed is neither a
plant nor animal, but another form of organism altogether. Seaweed is
similar to a plant in that it uses pigments, such as chlorophyll, to synthesize food through photosynthesis. Seaweed contains vitamins, minerals, polysaccharides (a type of sugar), and antioxidants, all of which
can be harvested from this natural resource. Seaweed exists in nature
as brown, red, and blue-green varieties. These color variations occur because each contains its own unique pigment that is capable of absorbing light, which is used as an energy source for photosynthesis.

Brown Algae. Brown algae are perhaps the best studied of all algae
species. Brown algae contain polyphenolic antioxidants and polysaccharides. These elements have been shown to prevent protein glycation, reduce inflammation and offer wrinkle-busting benefits by

inhibiting collagen and elastin breakdown. The polysaccharides block AGE formation and reduce its buildup in tissues by blocking receptors for AGEs. While you find won't specific ingredients such as the names of the polyphenols or polysaccharides listed on a cosmeceuticals label, you will find algae extract listed. One of the most valuable types of brown algae is the species *Ecklonia* (also known as kelp or cava). Studies have shown that *Ecklonia* is chock-full of healthy ingredients that make it a go-to for those in the know.

Red Algae. Red algae get their brilliant color from powerful antioxidants called carotenoids. You may have heard of the antioxidant astaxanthin that is harvested from the red algae *Haematococcus pluvialis*. This antioxidant has been shown to be 550 times more powerful than vitamin E and 6,000 times more powerful than vitamin C. Look out, free radicals! Astaxanthin also protects skin from damaging UV rays, especially those long wavelength UVAs that age your skin. It inhibits collagen and elastin breakdown and puts the brakes on UV pigmentation. By now, we're sure you won't be surprised when we tell you that astaxanthin also inhibits protein glycation, making it a winner on our list of all-stars.

Other Important Glycation Inhibitors

Although these ingredients do not come from plants or the sea, they are naturally occurring antioxidants found in the body. Alpha lipoic acid and L-carnosine are well known for their ability to prevent glycation and protect against free radicals. For this reason, they are included in our list of all-star ingredients.

Alpha Lipoic Acid (ALA)

Alpha lipoic acid is a nonenzymatic antioxidant that scavenges free radicals and reduces oxidative stress. Scientific studies have demonstrated that collagen abnormalities, including collagen cross-linking and reduction of collagen production caused by a high-sugar diet, can be

SWEET SUCCESS
Emily

Emily, a forty-four-year-old housewife with three teenage kids, was looking for a new look and a treatment plan to gain a more youthful appearance. Her main complaints were facial redness, puffiness, and fine lines and wrinkles. She just looked older than her years. Dr. Farris explained to Emily that she had a mild case of rosacea, which is common in women her age. She had tried lots of over-the-counter solutions and admitted to being a home shopping beauty junkie. When she arrived at Dr. Farris's office, she was toting a bag full of products she had purchased with a receipt that far exceeded her results. What she really needed was a mommy makeover that included weight loss, good skin care, and a sensible workout regimen. Much to her surprise, Dr. Farris examined her diet before she looking at her bag of skin-care goodies. Dr. Farris explained how dietary sugar affects skin negatively, causing inflammation that can leave skin looking prematurely aged. She then detoxed Emily's skin-care regimen, removing all the complicated, expensive, and unnecessary steps and merchandise, and started her on the Sugar Detox regimen for both diet and skin care. One month later, Emily returned for a follow-up visit. She had lost 9 pounds, but even more important was the change in her face. Her skin was far less red than before she had started the program. Her husband had commented on the change. "He usually doesn't notice anything," she remarked, "but even he said that I look younger." Dr. Farris saw a big improvement in Emily's rosacea, which was now barely visible, and a brightness to her skin that made it more radiant. Emily remains committed to staying on the maintenance plan for both her dietary and skin-care needs.

avoided by supplementation with alpha lipoic acid. Cosmeceuticals containing alpha lipoic acid have also been studied. When women used a 5 percent alpha lipoic acid cream on half of their face for twelve weeks, they saw improvement in skin roughness and appearance, when compared to the side treated with a cream that did not contain alpha lipoic acid. This potent antioxidant is a promising option for treating aging skin and reducing skin glycation.

L-Carnosine

L-carnosine, a potent antioxidant that inhibits glycation, is widely available in supplement form and has been proposed as an anti-aging therapy. In a study reviewing the benefits of this oral supplement, women taking a carnosine supplement for three months saw an improvement in their skin's appearance, including a reduction in fine lines and wrinkles. L-carnosine is among the most popular ingredients in antiglycation cosmeceuticals. Studies have demonstrated that this dipeptide is effective at preventing skin glycation, making it an all-star in our book.

10

The Sugar-Exercise Connection

The Sugar Detox isn't just about food and skin care; exercise is also a huge component here. With help from top personal trainer Liz Barnet, we've created a fitness plan for everyone from a couch potato to a gym enthusiast.

Think about it this way: How often have you used sugar to bump your energy or had a sweet treat because you were feeling blue? Now that you've committed to overcoming your reliance on sugar, you'll find many other things—food and otherwise—will take the place of sugar in your life. Exercise is one of them. Physical movement is a great complement to the detox diet and an essential part to the program as a whole.

Okay, we've heard all the excuses before: You're too busy, or your knees have hurt ever since that skiing accident ten years ago, or even the worst excuse of all, you hate to exercise. We know it's hard to get started, but trust us: Once you get into the routine, you'll soon begin to see and feel the benefits that will keep you coming back. And don't worry—we're not going to get all boot camp on you.

Believe it or not, there is a physiological reason that exercise makes you feel good. Exercise releases endorphins—chemicals in your brain that cause that exhilarated feeling after a hard workout. Ever hear of the "runner's high"? Endorphins. Exercise is also a great stress reliever and can be used to counteract depression. And there's more good news: Exercise makes your skin look good. It increases blood flow to all tissues, including your skin, leaving you with a rosy afterglow. Exercise also helps with sagging skin, because toned muscles provide a better supporting structure for it. So we'll have no more complaining about flabby arms or sagging knees, okay?

Besides your feeling and looking good, there are also many health benefits to exercise, including weight loss; improved bone density; cardiovascular health; and lowered blood pressure, lipids, and yes, blood sugar. And a study from California Polytechnic State University found that a good, sweaty workout can actually slow down blood flow to the part of your brain that controls food intake, helping you ignore those pesky sugar cravings.

We are not going to overburden you with exercise, because we believe that once you get the sugar out of your diet, adding a little exercise becomes easy, creating a healthy cycle: As you start to feel better on the diet plan, you will want to exercise more. And as you look and feel even better overall, you will have the motivation to keep to your new, healthy habits.

Couch Potatoes Go Viral

In today's world, most of us sit, then sit, and then sit some more. We understand that you may spend hours at sedentary activities, both at work and home. Office work may keep you chained to your desk for hours on end. We also understand that once you get home, you might like to watch TV or videos or surf the net for still more hours. All of this inactivity gives new meaning to the term *couch potato*. We don't love potatoes in your diet—or as a description, either.

We spend way too much time on the computer and using other electronic devices that make life easier, and also make us lazier (with the advent of cell phones becoming an extension of our arm, we don't even have to get up off our fat behind to answer the phone!). There is overwhelming scientific evidence to support the notion that a sedentary lifestyle is hazardous to your health. It can lead to being overweight and to developing such diseases as metabolic syndrome and diabetes. A study of previously healthy adults who cut down their daily activity to sedentary levels showed that these individuals began immediately to have increased blood sugar spikes after meals. Sedentary adults also have higher fasting insulin levels—and higher insulin levels lead your body to continuously store fat. So suffice it to say that the combination of inactivity and a poor diet is causing a major health crisis that it is literally killing us.

Muscle Up to Control Blood Sugar

There are so many health benefits of regular exercise that entire textbooks have been written on the subject. Here, we are going to focus on how exercise can be used to control and lower blood sugar and why it's important for weight loss.

Carbohydrates are the fuel for the body. Organs such as the brain, skeletal muscle, heart, and liver, rely on carbohydrates as a source of energy when they need it. When blood sugar levels are high—for instance, after a meal loaded with carbohydrates—the body's insulin will signal organs to take up the glucose and store it as glycogen. Skeletal muscle stores about 80 percent of the body's glycogen because muscle makes up such a large portion of the body's mass. The liver is actually filled with more glycogen ounce for ounce as compared to muscle, but it is a much smaller organ so it doesn't contain nearly as much. The brain and heart store smaller quantities of glycogen. When your muscles contract during exercise, they use glycogen for fuel. As the stored glycogen depletes within the muscle fibers, the muscles begin to fatigue. After exercise, your muscles immediately begin to take up more glucose, turning it into glycogen to replace what was lost during exercise. The other interesting thing is, the more you exercise, the more sensitive your muscles become to insulin and the more glycogen your muscles can store. So if you participate in sports or exercise on a regular basis, you have an increased capacity to store glycogen, giving your muscles more energy and stamina. This is why sports conditioning and training is so important. It is this continuous cycle of glycogen production and glycogen depletion in your muscles that makes exercise such an important factor in blood sugar control. Exercise helps your body store carbohydrates and utilize glucose in a healthy way.

Small Changes, Big Results

Even if you fall on the couch potato end of the spectrum, you can make an immediate improvement—without even going to the gym or even getting on your treadmill at home—simply by increasing your daily physical activity. By definition, physical activity is any type of movement, period. To increase your physical activity, all you have to do is start doing such things as using the stairs instead of the elevator. If you drive to the mall, park a little farther from the entrance, just to walk a bit.

Scientific studies have shown that just taking short breaks from sedentary activities can improve glucose metabolism and lower blood sugar. Something as simple as getting up and standing or walking for just five minutes every hour will do the trick. Taking breaks from sedentary activity will jump-start weight loss, prevent weight gain, and even reduce your risk for diabetes. Doctors treating patients with diabetes and metabolic syndrome now routinely recommend increasing daily physical activity. Diabetics who take more frequent breaks from sedentary activity see health benefits, including smaller waistlines, lower triglyceride levels and lower postmeal glucose levels.

Increasing physical activity is such an easy thing to do, and it will come back to you in terms of health benefits almost immediately.

8 Easy Ways to Increase Movement Every Day
1. Take the stairs instead of the elevator.
2. Walk to a co-worker's desk instead of sending an e-mail.
3. Park a block farther away.
4. Do nearby errands on foot, instead of getting back into the car to drive separately to each of them.
5. Take 5 minutes between projects to stretch.
6. Get off the bus or subway one stop earlier.
7. Perform simple exercises in your office (squatting to your chair, pushups against wall or desk, tricep dips from chair)
8. Find ways to increase your steps instead of multitasking to reduce them.

Cardio and Resistance Training

Adding a more dedicated exercise routine to your lifestyle is going to take a little more effort than just increasing physical activity, but we promise not to make it too painful. By "exercise routine," we mean planned, structured, and repetitive activities that are done to improve your physical fitness, strength, and endurance. The current federal recommendation is 150 minutes a week of moderate-intensity exercise or 120 minutes a week of high-intensity exercise. Now, if those numbers seem daunting, let's break it down into thirty-minute increments. To meet these goals, you could do a half-hour of moderate exercise five times a week or more intense exercise four times a week. If that seems too hard for you, you can break it down even more, into fifteen minutes in the morning and fifteen in the afternoon or evening, or even into ten minutes three times a day.

Any complete exercise program should include both resistance training and cardiovascular exercise. These types of exercise do two very different things for your body, and both are important for good health and for controlling glucose metabolism. A combination of cardiovascular exercise plus weight training has been shown to be the ideal exercise to help you reduce your risk of type 2 diabetes.

Cardiovascular exercise (a.k.a. cardio), as the name implies, gets the blood pumping, raises your metabolism, and improves cardiovascular health. Increasing your metabolism helps you burn calories even while at rest or sleeping and enables you to use food more efficiently. Cardiovascular exercise is characterized by repetitive movements that use your whole body. Cardio can be anything from walking to running, stair climbing, dancing or skating, or engaging in sports.

Resistance, or strength, training is pretty much what it sounds like, too: It is any type of exercise during which the muscles contract against external resistance, either by using your own body weight or by adding weights as you work out. This type of movement increases strength, tone, and muscle mass. Resistance training also helps improve bone mass, making it particularly important for women who are at risk for osteoporosis.

Here is more about how cardio and resistance exercise could work for you.

Cardio

The most basic things you are trying to achieve during cardio are strengthen your heart, specifically, and become more physically fit, in consequence and in general. When you begin to exercise, the first thing you will notice is your heart beating faster as it tries to deliver more blood—and thus, oxygen—to the muscles, helping them make energy needed to sustain the movement. The blood also removes waste products such as carbon dioxide and lactic acid, which builds up during exercise. With repeated exercise, your heart becomes stronger, allowing it to be more efficient at delivering blood to the rest of your body.

When you exercise, you will also notice that you are breathing harder and faster. This is because those waste products signal the respiratory center in your brain to tell your respiratory muscles to work harder. You may recall from grade school science class that you breathe in oxygen and exhale carbon dioxide—this mirrors what your red blood cells are actually doing throughout your body. With increased respiration, your lungs fill up with much-needed oxygen that is then carried to the muscles by your blood cells via a protein called hemoglobin. When they reach your muscles, the hemoglobin doesn't go back empty. Instead, it deposits the precious oxygen into your muscles, picking up the above-mentioned waste products, especially carbon dioxide, and brings those back to the lungs. Back at home base, the hemoglobin gives up its load of carbon dioxide and picks up more oxygen to take back to your muscles. This cycle repeats itself over and over again. So, don't think of it as panting—all that deep breathing is a good thing! The more oxygen your body is capable of processing through your respiratory system, the more efficiently your muscles will work; and the more calories you burn, the stronger they will become. Of course, the more you exercise, the more efficient this entire system becomes.

As noted earlier, walking, hiking, jogging, or running; biking; jumping rope; swimming; and, of course, such active sports as tennis all qualify as cardio. Cross-country skiing and snowshoeing are great winter cardio options for the outdoor enthusiast. Newer forms of cardio such as Zumba or hip-hop, cardio-boxing, or spinning are tons of fun. Pick something you feel comfortable with and build your endurance and cardiovascular fitness slowly. Note: If you suffer with any type of joint problem, you are better off choosing a low-impact type of cardio such as swimming or biking.

It's important that you start exercising slowly and not overexert yourself (if you're just starting out, just make sure to seek out a beginner-level class). Remember, slow and steady wins the race in the end. The goal is not to overwork your body, but to build up endurance gradually over time. Stick with the program for at least four weeks, or the 31-days of the Sugar Detox, and you will start seeing amazing changes in both your body and your endurance.

Endurance, which is a series of adaptive physiologic responses that happen over a period of time as a result of regular exercise, increases your stamina and allows you to exercise for longer periods of time, increasing your overall fitness. Within weeks after beginning an exercise routine, your heart will begin to pump more efficiently, allowing you to be able to handle your workouts without causing your heart rate to go so high. Your body will begin to be able to deliver more oxygen to the muscles being used, and this will bring your breathing rate down as that oxygen is delivered to muscles more efficiently. Also, your muscles will begin to store more glycogen, allowing you to work out for longer periods of time. Endurance is what you are striving for as you become more physically fit. But remember, it doesn't happen overnight. You have to build it slowly, one step at time.

Note: Before beginning any type of cardiovascular workout that increases your heart rate, you should consult with your physician.

Resistance Training

Resistance, or strength, training is often an overlooked component of exercise. Everyone loses muscle mass with age: From about the age of forty-five, the average person loses muscle mass at the rate of about 1 percent per year, rising to about 2 percent from the age of fifty. Resistance training is the best way to increase muscle mass and overall strength. It also helps you perform daily activities with a lower risk of injury. You will be less likely to suffer a fall, and overall more likely to remain independent and self-sufficient as you age.

Also, sculpted muscles make you look better! Often, women are afraid of weight training for the fear of becoming too muscular. That's not the case, as women don't produce enough testosterone on their own to truly "bulk up." Sculpted and well-defined muscles make skin appear tauter, reducing the appearance of cellulite and sagging skin. And don't forget that increasing muscle mass helps you burn calories, as the more muscle you have, the more calories you burn, even when you aren't being active. That's all good! While muscle definition takes awhile to start showing (and, due to the differences in hormonal makeup and muscular structure, women have a more difficult time than men when it comes to gaining and maintaining sufficient muscle mass), what goes on behind the scenes starts happening immediately. Like cardio, resistance training improves glucose metabolism, helps control blood sugar, and improves insulin sensitivity.

Now that you understand the basics, let's get off that couch and get started on your Sugar Detox exercise regimen.

Calculating Your Target Heart Rate

To maximize exercise benefits, you need to make sure that you are working your heart rate in the appropriate zone. Learning your target heart rate and keeping it in this range while you exercise is the best way to ensure you're exercising safely and effectively.

The first thing you need to do is calculate your **maximum heart rate**, which can be obtained by a simple formula: 220 minus your age. There are more complicated ways to find a more accurate maximum heart rate, but this is the easiest way for you to get an approximation. For example, if you are forty years old, 180 beats per minute is your maximum heart rate (220 − 40 = 180). This is the upper limit of your target heart range, depending on your experience and health situation.

Your **target heart rate** (THR) range lies somewhere between 50 and 75 percent of your maximum heart rate. This is the range you want to remain in for the majority of exercise, to ensure you are challenged safely. To obtain your target heart rate, multiply your maximum heart rate by 0.5 (50 percent) for the low end, and then calculate the upper range by multiplying your maximum heart rate again, this time by 0.75 (75 percent). Using our example, for a maximum heart rate of 180 beats per minute, the THR would be 90 to 135 beats per minute (180 × 0.5 = 90; 180 × 0.75 = 135). According to the American Heart Association, this is considered a safe range for your heart rate during your exercise routine.

By keeping your heart rate within this range, you will safely burn calories without overexerting; you can also learn how to judge how hard you're working and see improvements over time. You can monitor your heart rate while exercising by simply placing your index and middle fingers (don't use your thumb) over the inside part of your wrist and counting how many beats occur in ten seconds, then multiply that by six. This will give your heart rate per minute. Many cardio exercise machines have a feature that can determine your heart rate, or you can even buy a simple heart rate device at any sports store or online.

Exercise 101: Getting Started

The hardest part about exercising is finding—or making—the time to do it! But those who make exercising a part of their daily routine are the ones who are most likely to stick to it and have success. The trick is to dedicate a small and regular allotment of time to workouts, just the same as you might not even think twice about never missing your favorite half-hour TV show.

If you have a super busy work schedule, it might be best to exercise first thing in the morning. This way you have completed your exercise before the activities of the day begin, plus it's less likely that something will come up that will get in the way of your workout. If you have kids to get off to school, then working out at lunchtime or even after work might be better. After all, workouts are great stress relievers and can help you put the worries of the day behind you. If you travel for work, get in the habit of taking your workout clothes with you so that you can keep your routine consistent (you can always travel with a favorite exercise DVD or video loaded onto your laptop, for workouts in your hotel room; some hotels even offer the amenity of a workout room free of charge to paying guests).

If you are new to exercise, we understand you might be a little intimidated to join a gym right away. While you may think gyms are only full of toned and sculpted models, the truth is that they serve people of all shapes and sizes—and chances are, you'll meet someone else who is just starting out, too. If you're not ready to take the membership plunge, then we recommend that you start by using a combination of at-home and outdoor activities. (A park is a great place to get some cardio while enjoying the outdoors.)

Before beginning your cardio, make sure you buy a good pair of walking or running shoes that fit well. Dermatologists treat lots of foot problems, including blisters and calluses, caused by improperly fitting shoes. You can also damage your toenails if your shoes don't provide you with some cushion and room in the toe box. Make sure your socks are snug and not too bulky. If you are going to do your cardiovascular exercise outdoors, don't forget sunscreen and a hat. Schedule your outdoor workouts early in the morning or after four o'clock in the afternoon. Avoiding the peak rays of the sun will keep your skin looking good and reduce your risk of developing skin cancer.

For resistance workouts, you will need just a few simple tools that can be purchased in any major discount retail store or online: An exercise mat is a must-have item that can be purchased almost anywhere. It's also a great idea to pick up a couple of light dumbbell weights as well: 3 pounds if you are a beginner, to as much as 10 pounds if you are more advanced.

Putting Your Heart into It—Your Cardio Regimen

Beginners-Level Cardio

Beginners should start with thirty minutes of mild to moderate-level cardio at an intensity that keeps your heart rate within the target zone. Choose whatever type of cardiovascular exercise appeals to you. The easiest cardio to do is simply to walk at a brisk pace. Study after study has shown that a good, fast walk improves cardiovascular health and stimulates weight loss. Keep yourself engaged by listening to music on headphones. Challenge yourself by seeing how fast you can walk briskly to a goal, such as a street lamp or corner. If you find a walking buddy, that could also help the time pass while keeping you both motivated. At your workplace, you can get in some cardio by taking a break and walking up and down a flight of stairs a few times. If you prefer exercising at home, plenty of shows on television and the Internet feature fitness gurus doing cardio workouts. Pick one you like and join in for thirty minutes. Exercise videos are also great and make it even more convenient for you to fit in your cardio workout.

Cardio should be done at least three days a week. That said, true beginners should start with twenty minutes of cardiovascular activity. If that's too much to start, aim for just ten minutes—but try to do something every day. This will help your body adjust to all the new activity. Once you reach the twenty-minute threshold with ease, add one more minute to your workout per workout until you reach thirty minutes. This will be your new baseline for slow and steady cardio. You don't have to do thirty minutes at once; you can break it up into two fifteen-minute workouts spread throughout the day. As you become more fit, increase your cardio workouts to four or five times a week.

Moderate to Advanced Cardio

If you've been exercising regularly, it may be time to kick it up a notch. One way you can do this is by lengthening the duration of your cardio workout. For example, if you normally do thirty minutes a day, try increasing by two-minute increments per workout or every other work-out, working up to sixty minutes. This increased time will push you to become more physically fit and improve endurance. It is important as you increase your time and intensity that you closely monitor your heart rate, making sure to keep it in the target zone.

You can also increase the intensity of your cardio workout. Add some hills to your walk or run or bike ride. One of the advantages to working out in a gym is that the equipment allows you to increase the intensity easily: treadmills can be set to simulate walking uphill by increasing the incline; bikes and cross-trainers have similar built-in ways to increase resistance.

An additional benefit to going to a gym is that most of them have a variety of workouts, such as boot camp, spin class, and aerobic danc-ing. These are excellent for more advanced cardio training—and they're just plain fun! The secret to successful cardio training is finding some-thing you love to do and sticking to it.

High-Intensity Training

Perhaps you have heard of high-intensity training (HIT). Although this type of exercise isn't for everyone, it's important to cover this topic in this chapter. HIT is a low-volume, high-intensity workout that is popu-lar because it saves time and gets quick results. In this type of workout, you do bursts of high-intensity cardio for a set period of time, alternat-ing with rest periods. For our purposes, that burst of high-intensity car-dio is one minute. For example, a workout might be to sprint on a bike or run at maximum speed for one minute, followed by at least a minute of recovery time, repeated for a total of ten to twenty minutes. Even try-ing for quick bursts for twenty seconds and then resting for ten sec-onds, in a total of eight rounds, will give you four minutes of great HIT.

Studies have shown that HIT can be used to improve fitness, increase endurance, and lower blood sugar. High-intensity training is an advanced form of exercise and should be used only under the guidance of your physician and a professional trainer. But even if you aren't the most phys-ically fit, you can still benefit from a modified version of HIT. For example, if you have been doing the same half-mile walk a few times a week, try to kick it up a notch: Without going to any extremes, adjust your high-intensity intervals to be slightly above your usual intensity, while remembering that they need to be done in very short bursts interspersed with a rest longer than each burst. For example, if you walk, try to jog for thirty to sixty seconds, then rest for one to two minutes. If you're comfortable with jogging, try running for thirty seconds or sprinting for fifteen seconds, followed by a minute or half-minute rest, respectively. The most important rule of thumb is, the higher the intensity, the shorter the interval and the longer the recovery period. This will ensure you are challenging yourself in a safe and effective way.

If you aren't comfortable increasing your speed, switch up what you're doing. Take a break during your workout to throw in some jumping jacks, or drop and do a few push-ups, or even get down and hold a plank position as long as you can. Varying the speed or the intensity of your workout will challenge your body and keep it guessing. Just as your mind can get bored of the same old workout, your body can get bored and plateau as well, which can lead to your becoming inattentive to good form. These are all safe and attainable ways to keep your heart rate up, prevent you from plateauing, and increase your results.

Get Pumped, Burn Fat—Your Resistance-Training Workout

Although most of us think of weight training as a guy thing, women need strength (resistance) training just as much as, if not more than, men do. It's a fact that as you age, you lose muscle mass. Decreased muscle leads to a decreased metabolic rate, which means you are more likely to store extra calories as fat. Of course, that's the last thing you want to happen. Dr. Farris sees patients every day who are looking for a laser or other quick-fix device for removing unwanted fat. Some complain of tummy fat, while others obsess about their thighs. What these patients don't realize is that they don't need a doctor to remove unwanted fat. By embracing the weight room, they can take advantage of the ultimate fat burner: their own body weight! Although thirty minutes of cardio burns more calories than thirty minutes of resistance training, the latter allows you to continue burning calories even after your workout is over—which means it burns more calories overall. This is because muscle is more metabolically active than fat and requires more calories and energy. A pound of muscle requires 50 calories a day to sustain it, meaning that muscle is burning calories even when you are resting. The good news is that you can build muscle at any age by engaging in some type of resistance training or simply lifting weights. (Note: If you are a novice at the latter, ask a professional trainer to demonstrate how to do it properly.)

As noted earlier, resistance training is designed to work your muscles in a progressive way, using your own body weight or small added weights as you do squats, lunges, and push-ups. Each muscle group is worked individually with a set of repetitive movements (reps). Basic resistance training should work the biceps, triceps, shoulders, back, chest, abdomen, gluteal muscles, thighs, and calf muscles. It's important to understand that you cannot lose fat in a specific place by weight training. That's why doing sit-ups or crunches won't magically melt away tummy fat, and lifting your legs while wearing ankle weights won't slim your thighs. Working all the various muscle groups in your body will increase overall muscle mass, which will in turn make your body a more efficient fat-burning furnace. The most efficient way to approach strength training is by targeting the larger muscle groups; the more muscles you use at once, the more calories you will burn overall.

Choose Your Own Adventure—But Be Smart!

Here are few basics you should consider before you begin the resistance-training exercises that follow. Keep in mind that the goal of a particular exercise should be to properly execute that exercise with good form and enough resistance to impose a challenge on the muscles. Sometimes your own body weight might be sufficient, as in a push-up or a squat, and sometimes you may need to add an external load in the form of a weight. For our purposes, you should have access to a set of 5-pound and 10-pound dumbbells; but if you are an absolute beginner, you may want to invest in a set of 3-pound weights as well. A resistance band is also helpful for certain modifications of exercises and just to mix things up.

It is important to balance the amount of work you are doing with an appropriate amount of rest time, just as with cardiovascular training. It is helpful to think of strength training exercises in terms of repetitions (reps) and sets. A repetition is doing a particular exercise to completion once, with good form all the way through. A set is a certain number of repetitions strung together, one after the other. We suggest that for any particular exercise, you should aim to complete 8 to 12 reps with good form per set, and to complete at least 2 to 3 sets per workout. This particular breakdown of reps and sets is most useful for general health and fitness, modest improvements in strength, and position changes in physique.

To judge whether you are using the correct amount of weight for an exercise, you want the last couple of repetitions per set to feel difficult, particularly during your last set.

Basic Resistance (Weight) Training

Equipment. You'll need a set of weights, plus a mat or towel for the floor, and a chair or bench. Optional: inflatable exercise ball.

Clothing and Environment. You should wear comfortable clothing that's neither too loose nor too restrictive. Sneakers are fine for your feet. You can do these exercises anywhere—at the gym or in your own living room.

You can select from a vast majority of exercises that will get you results, but sometimes the simpler, the better. We have selected the following strength-training exercises because they are simple and yet effective, they recruit the largest muscle groups, and they are already recognizable to most people. There is a low risk for injury as long as you pay attention to proper form. You can manipulate certain variables (external load, exercise order, number of repetitions, rest periods) to constantly challenge your body in new ways while still sticking to this exercise selection.

For each exercise, we provide the setup and instructions for the basic version of the exercise, plus intermediate and advanced options.

Squat

The squat is an excellent total body toner; it recruits the largest muscles of the lower body, which in turn blasts major calories. Squats improve your form and strength in practically any physical activity, from bike riding, walking, skiing, dancing, hiking, to just getting up out of a chair. Squats help sculpt the legs and lift the booty!

Setup. Stand with your feet hip distance apart, toes facing straight forward or slightly turned out. The squat can be performed without weights (beginner), holding a weight in each hand with your arms by your sides (intermediate), or with a weight resting on each shoulder (advanced).

Exercise. With your upper body upright, start by bending your hips and knees and leading downward with your glutes (buttocks), as if you were sitting in an imaginary chair behind you. (For beginners or those with poor balance, you can and should use a real chair for support and guidance.) Inhale as you lower yourself until your thighs are parallel to floor, then exhale as you press back up to stand.

Note: Keep your spine tall and try not to pitch your torso forward over your thighs. Be sure not to round your upper back and or thrust your shoulders forward, especially if using weights. Watch to be sure your knees stay aligned with your toes and hips and don't collapse in toward each other.

Plank

The plank is the one exercise that every single person can and should include in his or her repertoire. Much more effective than crunches for toning the core muscles, the plank sculpts your muscles from head to toe, when executed properly. Rather than completing planks by repetitions, hold a plank with good form as long as you can, trying to increase your time during each workout.

Setup. For a high plank (which looks like the top of a push-up; see page 150), start with your feet hip distance apart, place your hands, shoulder distance apart, on the floor or a bench. Make sure your wrists, elbows, and shoulders are aligned. If you have wrist issues, you may make a fist with each hand and rest on your knuckles, or try the forearm plank, which has the same alignment as the high plank except that you are resting on your forearms and elbows (place your forearms flat directly under your shoulders, either running parallel or with your hands clasped so your arms make a V shape from elbows to wrists).

Exercise. Step backward with your legs raised from the floor so you are in a long, straight line from your shoulders to your feet. Breathing evenly and deeply, hold for as long as possible, aiming for at least 30 seconds to start. You may rest and restart as needed.

Note: It is very important to keep your abdominals engaged as you continue to breathe. Look down at the floor or your hands to keep your neck long and relaxed. Don't allow your hips to sag down or pop up. Imagine squeezing every muscle from your head to your toes.

Push-ups

Push-ups are an excellent upper-body and core strengthener, when properly executed. They are also an important movement for daily life, one that will help you when you need to push yourself out of bed or off the floor. Expect toned triceps and chest muscles as a result. This is especially helpful for ladies who are trying to fight the effects of gravity on the front of their body!

Setup. Place your hands slightly wider than shoulder distance apart either on a wall (beginner), a bench or counter (intermediate), or the floor, while holding a plank position (for advanced version; see the plank exercise for specific setup details). Alternatively, instead of placing your hands on an elevated platform, you can put them on the floor but assume a modified plank position on your knees instead of your feet. Be sure to keep your head aligned with your neck and look forward.

Exercise. Inhale as you bend your elbows to at least 90 degrees, lowering the body in one straight line. Exhale as you straighten your arms and return back to your starting position.

Note: Be sure to engage your core muscles by pulling your navel area toward your spine. Don't allow your hips to sag or your butt to pop up. Point your elbows straight out to the side for a traditional push-up; or keep them close to your body for a "yoga," or triceps, push-up. The latter may be easier for individuals with shoulder pathologies.

Row (or Pull)

It is important to counter every pushing exercise (such as the push-up) with at least one pulling action. This is because our sedentary lifestyle, such as sitting at the computer for long lengths of time, forces us into an uncomfortable, unattractive, hunched-forward position. If you find you have a lot of neck, shoulder, and back tension, be sure to add plenty of rowing or pulling motions, such as the ones mentioned next. They will improve your posture, combat back flab, and reduce the risk of injury.

Setup. Rows can be done using bands, cables, or free weights. To set up a row using a band or cable machine, anchor the band or cable slightly below shoulder height; you will be pulling horizontally, parallel to the floor. Another option is to set the anchor up high above you, so you will be pulling downward on a diagonal. These two setups work slightly different muscles and are both useful. To use free weights, stand with your torso angled forward about 45 degrees from the floor (individuals with lower back issues may want to avoid this setup). In either case, keep the knees and hips slightly bent and soft; the spine, long and straight; and the core, engaged.

Exercise. Starting with straight arms, exhale as you squeeze your shoulder blades together and bend your arms back, leading with the elbows. Inhale as you straighten your arms and return to start.

Note: Be sure to not let your shoulders creep up toward the ears in any of the positions. The abdominals should stay engaged to support the lower back. For beginners, keep your elbows close to the sides of the body as you pull back. For a more advanced variation, take the elbows wide as you pull back, in the same path as you would a push-up.

Lunge

There are many variations of the lunge, but it is essential to perfect your form in the basic versions before advancing to more complicated ones. Lunges are especially helpful for improving balance, as your legs are doing two different things at one time and are not positioned side by side. Like squats, lunges recruit all the muscles of the lower body and are therefore essential for increasing lean muscle mass, which will burn calories and give you definition.

Setup. Start with your feet parallel, hip distance apart. With one leg, take a step forward about a foot or so in front of you. For beginners, maintain this foot position, known as a split stance, to execute stationary lunges.

Exercise. Inhale as you bend both knees, trying to get them both to 90 degrees. Exhale as you straighten both legs to their starting position back together.

For the stationary lunge, your feet will remain in this split stance for all repetitions. The reverse lunge is an intermediate variation: Keeping one foot planted, step backward with the other foot and bend both knees before stepping forward back to start. The forward lunge is the advanced variation; keeping one foot planted, step the other foot forward as you bend both knees before stepping backward to start.

Note: It is very important to make sure that, whichever foot is the "front" foot, you distribute your weight over the heel of that foot. Putting too much body weight in the toes of the front foot (particularly during the forward lunge) will cause the heel to lift and put unnecessary pressure on the knee, making the lunge less effective. Whichever foot is in back, the heel will remain off the ground and the weight will be on the ball of the foot. Keep your torso tall and your abs engaged, no matter which variation you are completing. You can complete the lunge with or without additional weight.

Overhead Press

The overhead press is a great exercise for sculpting toned arms and shoulders while challenging your core strength. This is another variation of a push or a press, so be sure to counter it with a row or a pull.

Setup. Stand with your feet parallel and hip-distance apart. Hold a dumbbell in each hand at shoulder height, with your palms facing in. For a more advanced version, hold the dumbbells slightly to the outside of your shoulders, with your palms facing forward.

Exercise. Exhale as you press the weights overhead, inhale as you return to start. With the beginner version (palms facing in), the weights will go straight up and down. If your palms are facing forward, you will push the weights up in an arc shape until they touch overhead, before reversing the motion.

Note: Keep your hips and knees soft and bent, and your abdominals engaged, particularly when pressing overhead. Those with shoulder or lower-back issues may want to avoid this exercise.

Here is a basic chart to get you started in developing your own program. See page 158 for tips on incorporating this with cardio for a full week's worth of fitness.

TABLE 10.1 Developing Your Own Exercise Program

Exercise	Beginner	Intermediate	Advanced	Sets	Reps
Squat	To chair or bench, no weight	Weights held in hands, at sides, palms facing in	Elbows bent, weights resting on shoulders	3	8–12
Plank, on hands or elbows	Feet parallel and wide apart	Feet parallel and hip distance apart	Feet together or one foot up	2–3	15 seconds to start, working up to 30–90
Push-up	Knees on floor or standing with hands on wall	On an incline with hands on bench or counter	Full push-up position	2–3	5 to start; add 1 each workout; work up to 8–12
Lunge	Split stance (feet don't move)	Reverse lunge	Forward lunge	2–3 per leg	8–12
Row	Using band or cable, close grip (elbows in)	Bent over, close grip (elbows in)	Bent over, wide grip (elbows out)	3	8–12
Overhead press	Seated in chair with a back, close grip	Standing, close grip	Standing, wide grip	2–3	8–12

Don't Forget to Stretch

It's amazing how many people don't stretch before or after exercise. It's important not to start exercising without a minimum of a 5-minute warm-up period that should include some light stretching of the muscle groups you are going to work. In addition, the best time get a good stretch is after a workout, as muscles are more responsive to stretching once fully warmed up. After a workout of any kind, you should spend at least ten minutes stretching.

You don't have to do all of the following stretches, but make sure to target the ones that stretch the muscles you will use or have used in your workout. Here are some of our favorites:

Low Back Stretch. Lie on a mat or on the floor. With both knees bent and your feet flat on the floor, reach behind your knees with your hands and pull your feet off the mat. Hug your knees to your chest, pressing your back to the mat. This will give your lower back a good stretch. Hold for 15 seconds.

Hip and Gluteals. Lie on the mat with your knees bent, left foot on the floor, right ankle crossed on your left thigh just above the knee. Your legs will resemble the number 4. With both hands, reach around your left leg and gently pull your left knee up toward your body. Be careful not to overstretch—just enough to feel a little tension in your right hip and buttocks. Hold for 15 seconds and release. Repeat this stretch with your right leg on your left thigh.

Hamstring Stretch. To stretch the muscles on the back of your legs, start by lying down with your feet on the mat and your knees bent. Lift your right leg, with the leg straight and the knee slightly bent and your foot flexed. Reach down with both hands and grab just above the right knee, while keeping your hips on the mat. Gently pull the right leg toward your body until you feel a mild stretch on the back of your right thigh. Hold for 15 seconds and then repeat on the other side.

Abdominal Stretch. Lie facedown on your mat with your hands, palms down, directly under your shoulders, elbows bent and pointing upwards. Point your toes. Press into the mat as you extend your arms straight, keeping your head aligned with your spine, keeping your hips on the mat as you stretch the front of your torso. Exhale as you stretch your arms straight from mat to shoulder. Hold for 5 seconds and then repeat this stretch three times.

Shoulder and Upper Back Stretch. Kneel on the mat, sit your hips back onto your heels, and settle your body over your thighs. Extend your arms straight out in front of you pressing, down into the mat; your elbows should be straight; and your hands, palms down on the mat. Feel your shoulders and upper back stretch. Hold for 15 seconds.

Quadriceps Stretch. Lie on your left side, on the mat. Your left arm should be extended straight on the mat with your head and left ear resting on it. Keep your left leg straight and bend your right knee. Reach back with the right hand to grasp your right ankle and press your heel toward your buttocks. Pull only until you feel a mild tension in front of your thigh. Be very careful not to overstretch the knee. Hold for 15 seconds and then repeat on the other side.

Seated Inner Thigh Stretch. Sitting up on your mat, bend your knees and place the soles of your feet together. Try to have your feet positioned close to your body. With your hands on your knees, lean forward and press your knees down gently. Feel a mild tension in the inner thigh area. Hold for 15 seconds.

Calf Stretch. Standing about 12 inches away from a wall, place your forearms against the wall and lean forward. Step back with your right leg, keeping the leg straight, and press your right heel down. Feel a mild tension in the right calf. Hold for 15 seconds and then repeat on other side.

Chest Stretch. Either sitting or standing, extend your arms straight out to the side, with your palms forward. Relax your neck as you press your arms straight back. Hold, feeling a mild tension through your chest. Hold for 15 seconds.

Palm-Up Stretch. Either sitting or standing, extend your right arm out in front of your body, with your palm facing up. Grasp your right fingers with your left hand and gently pull your right fingers back and toward your body. Feel a mild tension in your right forearm. Hold 15 seconds and then repeat on other side.

Behind-Head Triceps Stretch. Either sitting or standing, drop your chin down to your chest and reach your right arm straight up overhead, palm forward. Bend your elbow and drop your right hand to the back of your neck (your palm will now face in). Reach overhead with your left arm and grasp just below your right elbow, gently pulling your right arm to the left. You should feel a mild tension in the back of your right upper arm. Hold for 15 seconds and then repeat on other side.

Standing Torso Side Reach. Stand with your feet at shoulder width, your toes pointing straight ahead. Place your right hand on your right hip for support, and reaching your left arm up and overhead, bend your torso to the right. Hold for 15 seconds and then repeat on the other side.

Neck Rolls. Begin by either sitting or standing. Drop your chin down to your chest. Keep your chin down close to your body and roll your neck from shoulder to shoulder in a smooth, controlled motion. Move your chin from side to side ten times.

The Sweet Spot

As we noted earlier, during the 3-Day Sugar Fix, it's best to not try anything new when it comes to exercise. Even those who exercise regularly should take it down a notch during this strict phase and stick to walking or light yoga or stretching.

Once Week 1 begins, you can increase your exercise. Following are some exercise plans, geared to various levels and experience.

Beginner. Two days per week light resistance training, 2 days per week cardio exercise. You can mix and match the resistance training and cardio during a workout, but still get moving at least four days per week. Include light HIT to build stamina. See Table 10.2 for an example.

TABLE 10.2 Exercises During the 3-Day Sugar Fix, Beginner

Sunday	Monday	Tuesday	Wednesday	Thursday	Friday	Saturday
20-minute walk: include five 1-minute speed walks, and 10 minutes of abdominals and thigh exercises.		40-minute walk; include ten 1-minute speed walks (or light jogging if you can handle it.)		Resistance training		20-minute walk; include five 1-minute speed walks or light jogs and light resistance training.

Intermediate. Two days per week resistance training, 2 days per week cardio exercise, with HIT. See Table 10.3 for an example.

TABLE 10.3 Exercises During the 3-Day Sugar Fix, Intermediate

Sunday	Monday	Tuesday	Wednesday	Thursday	Friday	Saturday
30-minute walk/run with five 1-minute speed increases. Follow with 15 minutes of resistance training.		Resistance training	45-minute aerobics class or video of your choice, e.g., spinning, Zumba, aerobic stepping, kickboxing.		30-minute walk/run with five 1-minute speed increases. Follow with 15 minutes of resistance training.	

Advanced. Two days per week resistance training, 3 days per week cardio exercise with HIT. See Table 10.4 for an example.

TABLE 10.4 Exercises During the 3-Day Sugar Fix, Advanced

Sunday	Monday	Tuesday	Wednesday	Thursday	Friday	Saturday
40-minute walk/run with ten 1-minute speed increases. Follow with 15 minutes of resistance training.	45-minute aerobic class or video of your choice.		Resistance training	45-minute aerobic class or video of your choice.		40-minute walk/run with ten 1-minute speed increases. Follow with 15 minutes of resistance training.

11

The Sweet Life:
Your Maintenance Plan

You've done it! The thirty-one days are over; and by the end of them, you're enjoying sugar in a healthy way through dairy, fruits, wine, chocolate, and the occasional dessert. Now you're probably wondering what the next steps are.

We ask you to adopt this maintenance plan as your permanent lifestyle. This allows you to have a little wiggle room to allow for special occasions, makes it somewhat easy to eat out in restaurants, and gives you flexibility to create your own meal plan that best suits your lifestyle. To help you further, we've included an entire chapter on Dining Out (see Chapter 12).

It really isn't hard to keep the principles of the plan in place long after you've finished the program.

Daily Maintenance Plan
Protein: minimum 3 servings (see page 7 for portion sizes)
Dairy: 2 servings, plus a splash in coffee if desired
Vegetables: unlimited quantity of approved veggies
Fruit: 1 apple + 1.5 servings of fruits
Fat: minimum 3 servings
Starch: 2 servings per day of approved starches + 1 serving of high-fiber crackers

Alcohol: maximum 5 glasses of red wine per week

Dessert: 1 ounce of dark chocolate (65% cacao minimum) daily; any other dessert besides dark chocolate will count as a starch and may occur twice a week.

It's important that you still keep things in check even though you're at your goal. The last thing we want you to do is to start to indulge and lose the progress that you worked so hard to achieve over the last thirty-one days.

Even by overeating something as healthy as fruit, the weight can start to creep back on and your sweet tooth will reappear. That's why we still limit your fruit choices and serving sizes. The maintenance plan optimizes the health benefits of fruit such as fiber, vitamins, minerals, antioxidants, and more, but without letting your sugar get out of hand.

While two servings of dairy may even seem generous at this stage of the game, remember how small the serving sizes are. So if you have a yogurt for breakfast and some cheese in your salad for lunch, then those are your dairy servings for the day.

Same thing for starches: Two servings plus crackers may seem like a lot on paper, until you realize that two slices of whole-grain bread equals two servings of starch.

How to Indulge

We're realists when it comes to how people eat and understand that you will come up against occasions to eat dessert or indulge in a food that isn't Sugar Detox approved. So we needed to come up with a way for people to be able to literally have their cake and eat it, too. Your twin aids to staying on track are planning ahead and making mindful decisions. During maintenance, you can include dessert up to twice a week—but for each dessert, you have to cross out one of your allotted starches. While, calorie for calorie or even nutrient for nutrient, this isn't an even exchange, as brown rice is clearly a healthier choice than chocolate mousse, it's a way of swapping sugar for sugar. Even more important, it's a way of forward thinking that's really important for any type of lifestyle maintenance. If you know you're going to any kind of event where you may be tempted to eat dessert, plan ahead and forgo that multigrain roll with your lunchtime salad. Or, if it comes upon you as a surprise—say, an office party you had not anticipated—skip one starch during the next twenty-four hours. It's that simple.

If You're Going to Go for It . . .

This may seem surprising coming from us, but if you're going to go for dessert—really go for it. By this we mean don't get the sorbet, opt for ice cream instead. There are a few reasons why we say this. First, non-fat desserts are simply loaded with sugar and contain nothing to help you digest it in a civilized way. Second, if you have prepared for dessert as just described, then don't feel guilty about indulging. You are compensating for it within the greater picture of a day's worth of acceptable foods. We want you to enjoy everything that you eat, so if you're eating that sorbet while you're staring longingly at the ice cream, then the sorbet isn't going to be nearly as satisfying and you'll end up with a small sugar high that's not even worth it. Eat the ice cream!

Mind and Body

One of the most important parts of the Sugar Detox is that this is a lifestyle, not a diet. That's one of the reasons why we mapped out the book the way we did: starting with all the amazing foods we want you to be eating instead of focusing on all the foods you shouldn't be having. By the end of the plan, the way you're eating shouldn't feel restrictive. It should feel normal, healthy, and balanced, with wiggle room to indulge when you want and a way to clean up or prepare when necessary.

Keeping to the maintenance plan shouldn't be difficult for you at all at this stage. Let's not forget how hard you worked during the 3-Day

Sugar Fix or even how hard Week 1 was! If you get off track, don't let it throw you into a sugar tailspin. Restart eating the right way at the immediate next meal. If you need another push, don't be afraid to tighten up your eating and start back on the earlier weeks (even trying the 3-Day plan again) to help you get back on track or to help push you toward your new goal. You've done it and we're proud of you. And that is as sweet as it gets!

Part Four

A **Place**
AT THE **Table**

12

How to Dine Out

Of course, there are going to be many occasions when you're eating out with friends or family. Here's a handy list of Sugar Detox–approved dishes and meals at the most popular kinds of restaurants. You'll see that some of the suggestions have particular weeks noted next to them; dishes without designated weeks are okay at any time during the plan.

In all cases, try to avoid menu items that involve frying, grilling, or roasting as their method of preparation. Many restaurants these days are mindful of special diets and do provide delicious alternatives.

Be mindful of portion sizes. If you are already using the plan at home, you should be able to judge, for example, how large a 6-ounce portion of protein appears. Don't be shy about divvying up your order on the plate to the correct meal size *as soon as it is served*, eating only that portion, and asking the staff to pack up the rest for you to take home. Or, if you know servings at an establishment are large, ask your dining companion to split an entrée with you. At a buffet, fill your plate once with the right proportions of food, and instead of going back for seconds, enjoy a glass of water or a cup of tea. Oh, and that reminds us: One of the best dining-out aids we know is to be sure to drink a large glass of water with a big squeeze of lemon before you even get down to eating, to fill you up with a refreshing burst of zero calories.

American

Bars and Grills

Order a broth-based soup or a salad, which are almost always available. Start off with shrimp cocktail or veggie crudités rather than a fried appetizer. A steak with steamed or roasted veggies on the side is a safe bet.

Opt For

Broth-based vegetable soup
Bun-less, cheese-less burger over a salad
House or garden salads, with grilled chicken, salmon, or shrimp
Open-faced sandwich on whole wheat bread (Week 4+)
Shrimp cocktail
Veggie crudités

Skip

Beer
Burgers, except as above
Potatoes (French fries, mashed, baked, etc.)
Fried appetizers (mozzarella sticks, potato skins, Buffalo wings, nachos, etc.)
Pizza
Sugary cocktails (piña coladas, margaritas, daiquiris)

Diners and Cafés

Diner and café menus are often laden with deep-fried foods and sugary treats, but there are plenty of options available. Salads are always a good choice; just make sure to order dressing on the side, or opt for oil and vinegar to avoid a sugary dressing. You can order dishes without a starch; for example, a turkey burger wrapped in lettuce, or poached eggs with spinach rather than with toast and/or potatoes.

Opt For

½ cup cantaloupe or ½ grapefruit (Week 2+)

Cottage cheese or plain yogurt (Week 1+)

Greek salad with grilled chicken, oil, and vinegar (feta Week 1+; omit grape leaves)

Green salad with oil and vinegar

Omelet with vegetables (you may add cheese Week 1+)

Plain oatmeal (Week 3+)

Poached eggs over spinach, with Canadian or turkey bacon

Turkey BLT (in a lettuce wrap Week 1+, or open-faced Week 4+)

Whole wheat, rye, or pumpernickel bread (Week 4+)

Skip

Burgers, unless served "on the plate" without cheese

Cheese (during 3-Day)

Coleslaw

Dressings that contain added sugar, including ketchup

Flavored or fruited yogurt

Dishes with cheese/white sauces (mac and cheese, chicken à la king)

Pasta

Potatoes (French fries, hash browns, home fries, mashed, baked)

Potpie, shepherd's pie, quiche, or other entrées with a crust

Tuna, potato, and pasta salads

White bread, bagels, rolls, muffins, and pastries

Steakhouse

Steakhouses have Sugar Detox–friendly options; just make sure to substitute roasted or steamed veggies or a salad for the potatoes that often accompany steak entrées. Sirloin and filet mignon are the leanest options.

Opt For

Cucumber and tomato salad

Filet mignon (6 ounces)

Green salad with oil and vinegar

Grilled fish or shellfish (lobster, shrimp, scallops)

Green salad
Lamb loin chops
Raw appetizers (oysters, tuna tartare, beef carpaccio)
Sautéed veggies
Steamed artichoke

Skip
The breadbasket
Burgers, except "on the plate" without cheese
Dressings, cocktail sauce, steak sauce, and ketchup
Fried fish or seafood
Pasta
Potatoes (French fries, mashed, baked)

Asian

Chinese

Order dishes steamed with sauce on the side, as often ingredients are flash-fried before sautéing. Steaming will ensure that doesn't happen. Soups are safe, as most of them are thin and vegetable-based, or made with chicken broth. Ask that no sugar or cornstarch be added to your dishes.

Opt For
Brown rice (Week 4+)
Chicken and vegetables with black bean sauce
Curried chicken and vegetables
Egg drop soup
Hot and sour soup
Mixed vegetables
Moo goo gai pan (chicken and mushrooms)
Sesame oil or soy sauce, for dipping
Steamed moo shu dishes without hoisin sauce or grain-based wraps
    (Use lettuce leaves or eat without wrapping.)
Steamed tofu, chicken, or shrimp

Skip
Dim sum
Dumplings and potstickers
Fried appetizers (egg/spring rolls, fried noodles, scallion pancakes,
    shrimp chips, shrimp toast, fried wontons, crab rangoons)
Fried or breaded entrées (e.g., General Tso's)
Noodle dishes (lo mein, mei fun, chow fun, noodle soups)
Sweet-and-sour, plum, or hoisin sauce
White or fried rice
Wonton soup

Indian

Vegetarian options abound in Indian restaurants. Take advantage of the
flavorful bean and lentil (dal) dishes. Order entrées without rice, potatoes (aloo) or breads (naan, poori, paratha). Avoid dishes with heavy
sauces (e.g., tikka masala, which includes cream). Some sauces are
coconut-, tomato-, or yogurt-based, which are fine.

Opt For
Brown rice (½ cup, okay Week 4+)
Channa masala
Chicken masala
Lentil (dal) entrées
Mulligatawny soup
Salted lassi (Week 1+)
Tandoori chicken, shrimp, or vegetables
Tikka masala
Saag paneer
Whole wheat roti (1 medium-size, okay Week 4+)

Skip
Fruit lassis
Korma
Pakoras

Rice dishes
Samosas

Japanese

Japanese restaurants have lots more to offer than tempura. Make sure to avoid rice (it is possible!), including in sushi. Sashimi is a great go-to and you can also opt for tataki: fish or meat that is briefly seared, then marinated with vinegar and served with ginger. Sip green tea.

Opt For
6 pieces sashimi
Beef negimaki, without sauce
Brown rice sushi roll (Week 4+)
Cucumber-wrapped roll (rice-free; a.k.a. naruto roll or cucumber sashimi roll)
Edamame
Green salad with rice vinegar and sesame oil
Miso soup
Sashimi handroll, without rice
Soba (buckwheat) noodles (½ cup, Week 3+)
Tartare
Tataki

Skip
Donburi
Ginger dressing
Ramen
Rice
Seaweed salad
Teriyaki sauce
Tonkatsu and other panko-breaded dishes

Korean

Korean sauces and marinades often include sugar, but if you opt for Korean barbecue you control the cooking and the sauce that goes on your food. For vegetarians, the tofu "steak" entrée is a popular choice, in addition to seafood.

Opt For
Brown rice (½ cup, Week 4+)
Buckwheat noodles (½ cup, Week 3+)
Grilled octopus
Korean barbecue (6 ounces of meats of choice)
Scallops
Seafood and vegetable stew
Soups without the noodles
Spicy tofu stew with seafood, eggs, or vegetables

Skip
Bibimbap and other rice dishes
Deep-fried or breaded dishes
Kimchi (unless no added sugar)
Marinades/sauces with added sugar
Noodle dishes (except as above)
Pancake-style appetizers

Thai and Vietnamese

Be careful when reading the menu at Thai or Vietnamese restaurants. Many dishes often come with noodles or rice, so be sure to ask your waiter any questions you may have. When ordering soups, ask to substitute vegetables for the noodles. Avoid fried tofu and ask for it steamed. Stay away from Thai or Vietnamese iced tea or coffee—both are made with way too much sugar.

Opt For
Chicken or shrimp lettuce wraps, no dipping sauce
Curry dishes, such as shrimp in coconut green curry
Dishes cooked with basil and chili sauce
Green papaya salad

Satay skewers without the dipping sauce (ask for soy and/or hot
  sauce instead)
Scallops
Seafood soup without the noodles (ask to substitute veggies)
Shrimp salad
Spring rolls made with lettuce instead of a rice flour wrap
Tom yum soup

Skip
Fried appetizers (e.g., Thai wontons or fried spring rolls)
Pho (noodle) soups
Rice dishes
Vermicelli, pad thai, and other noodle dishes
White, fried, or coconut rice

French

French cuisine brings two words to mind: *cheese* and *wine*. Thankfully,
you can have both in the later weeks; just keep an eye on portion sizes
and avoid rich cream sauces. Enjoy the flavorful meat, seafood, and vegetables without any guilt!

Opt For
Buckwheat crepes (Week 4+)
Coq au vin
Loin lamb chop or steak (6 ounces)
Lentil salad
Mixed greens with goat cheese (Week 1+)
Mussels in white wine and garlic
Niçoise salad, with olive oil and vinegar, omitting potatoes
Ratatouille
Small charcuterie/cheese board (Week 1+)
Whole wheat baguette (Week 4+)

Skip

Creamed soups

Creamy/cheesy sauces (béchamel, gratin)

Crepes (sweet or savory), except as above

Croissants

Frites

Pasta

White bread (baguettes) and pastries

Italian

Many Italian restaurants offer menu items besides pasta, including soups and salads, as well as seafood- and meat-based dishes. For an appetizer, try Italian wedding soup, steamed clams or mussels, tricolore salad, or antipasto (limit the cheese). As for entrées, order shrimp scampi and ask for a side of veggies in place of pasta. Order tomato sauce, garlic and olive oil, or clam sauce, rather than creamy Alfredo or vodka sauce.

Opt For

Antipasto platter

Caprese or tricolore salad (Week 2+)

Grilled calamari over greens with lemon juice

Italian wedding soup

Mixed seafood platter

Shrimp or chicken scampi, replacing pasta with greens

Steamed clams or mussels

Stracciatelle (Italian egg drop soup)

Whole wheat pasta (½ cup, Week 3+)

Skip

Calzone

Dishes with cheese sauce or breading (e.g., chicken parmigiana)

Italian or garlic bread, or focaccia

Pasta, except as above

Pizza

Polenta

Rice dishes

Mediterranean and Middle East

The Mediterranean diet is considered to be one of the healthiest in the world. Enjoy dishes originating from Greece, Turkey, and the Middle East. Ask for cucumber slices instead of pita bread to dip into sauces, and replace rice with a side salad.

Opt For

Greek salads with grilled chicken or fish and feta cheese (feta Week 1+)

Grilled fish, chicken, or shrimp kebabs

Haloumi or lebane (soft yogurt cheese) (Week 1+)

Mezze (hummus, baba ghanoush, taramsalata, with sliced veggies instead of pita)

Olives

Quinoa or bulgur tabbouleh (Week 3+)

Tomato or lentil soup (no sugar added)

Whole wheat pita (1 medium, Week 4+)

Skip

Couscous

Lavash and pita chips

White pita

White rice

Mexican

You can easily enjoy your favorite Mexican dishes with a few alterations. Instead of chips, dip crunchy jicama, bell pepper, or cucumber slices into guacamole or salsa. A lot of dishes come smothered in cheese and sour cream, so be on the lookout for those and request such accompaniments to be left on the side. Beans and rice is a popular dish; just ask for brown rice, if available, and choose black or pinto beans instead of refried beans.

Opt For
Burrito bowl (skip the tortilla)
Carne asada
Ceviche
Chicken, shrimp, or vegetable fajitas (skip the tortilla)
Grilled fish with salsa
Grilled veggies
Guacamole
Nopales (cactus leaves)
Tostada salad (without the shell)
Whole wheat tortilla, 1 small or ½ large (Week 4+)

Skip
Enchiladas
Flautas
Mole (the sauce is made with bread)
Nachos
Plantains
Quesadillas
Tacos

Spanish and South American

Spanish and South American restaurants have plenty of seafood options. Rice and potatoes are used frequently (we're looking at you, paella and croquetas) so make sure you speak to the waiter about what comes in your dish before you order. Often there are great tapas for everyone to share that include fish, olives, and vegetables.

Opt For

Avocado salad
Broquetas (beef skewers)
Ceviche
Cured anchovies or tuna
Dishes cooked in garlic and wine sauce
Gazpacho, without bread
Grilled squid or octopus
Mussels, shrimp, or lobster

Skip

Croquetas (croquettes)
Paella
Patatas bravas (potatoes)

13

Delicious, Easy
Sugar Detox Recipes

We want you to enjoy everything you eat while you're following the Sugar Detox. These recipes will encourage you to stick to the plan and savor every bite you take. All the recipes were developed or overseen by Chef Jason Brown, with a few contributions from guest chefs.

We've sorted the recipes by meal; each recipe has the nutritional information and the correct daily serving for the Sugar Detox plan, as well as a note telling you which week the recipe is for.

The Sugar Detox Trifecta

Everyone following the Sugar Detox plan should have these three key basic condiments in the kitchen. The spice blend can be used to season anything from popcorn to nuts to simple entrées; the vinaigrette makes any salad better; and the marinade turns simple proteins into a delicious meal!

Sugar Detox Spice Blend

MAKES ABOUT 4 TABLESPOONS SPICE MIXTURE

2 tablespoons dried rosemary
1 tablespoon dried sage
1 teaspoon ground ginger
½ teaspoon salt
½ teaspoon freshly ground black pepper

Mix all the ingredients together well. Use to season anything that you can think of!

Sugar Detox Vinaigrette

MAKES ABOUT 1½ CUPS VINAIGRETTE

1 recipe Sugar Detox Spice Blend
½ cup red wine vinegar
1 cup extra-virgin olive oil

In a cup or small bowl, whisk all the ingredients together until well combined. Store at room temperature in an airtight container.

Sugar Detox Marinade

MAKES ABOUT 1/2 CUP MARINADE

1 recipe Sugar Detox Spice Blend
¼ cup olive oil
Juice of 1 lemon
1 tablespoon lemon zest
1 clove garlic, minced

In a cup or small bowl, whisk together all the ingredients; pour over meat, seafood, or tofu; let sit for at least 30 minutes; cook; and enjoy!

Breakfast

Cottage Cheese–Oatmeal Pancakes

FOOD GROUP(S): 1 DAIRY, 1 STARCH
MEAL PLAN: WEEK 3

229.5 calories, 17.1 g carbohydrates, 7.2 g fat, 2.5 g saturated fat,
23 g protein, 2.1 g fiber, 531 mg sodium per serving

These pancakes are always a crowd-pleaser—so simple to make and yet still so delicious. Without any of those crazy sugar spikes you'd get from plain old pancakes, these keep you full and satisfied for hours. **SERVES 2**

1 cup low-fat cottage cheese
2 eggs
½ cup old-fashioned rolled oats

Combine all the ingredients and blend in a blender or food processor until smooth. Pour onto a nonstick skillet heated over medium to high heat and spread thinly. Cook until bubbling, about 2-4 minutes and flip over to cook for about 3 minutes on the second side, until done. Serve immediately.

Chia Pudding

FOOD GROUP(S): N/A
MEAL PLAN: 3-DAY

200 calories, 16.1 g carbohydrates, 11.6 g fat, 1.2 g saturated fat,
20 g protein, 13.5 g fiber, 24.5 mg sodium per serving

With a texture similar to that of fine tapioca, this no-cook pudding is filled with hearty chia seeds that have expanded into little pearls of yumminess! Make ahead of time or even the night before; it keeps in the refrigerator for up to three days. Have fun with experimenting with different seasonings, too, to spice it up. **SERVES 4**

2½ cups unsweetened almond or coconut milk

½ cup chia seeds

1 teaspoon vanilla extract

1 teaspoon ground cinnamon

Place all the ingredients in a bowl. Cover and refrigerate for at least 4 hours or overnight, stirring occasionally, until a puddinglike consistency is reached. Enjoy chilled.

Spinach-Egg Muffins

FOOD GROUP(S): N/A
MEAL PLAN: 3-DAY

104 calories, 3.4 g carbohydrates, 5.9 g fat, 2.6 g saturated fat, 7.5 g protein, 0.8 g fiber, 239.3 mg sodium per serving

Call them muffins, mini frittatas, or crustless quiches—whatever their name, these are the most convenient way to have eggs in the morning. Make the whole dozen and stick half in the freezer. Microwave them for one minute and you have an amazing hot breakfast! SERVES 6 (2 MUFFINS PER SERVING)

10 ounces frozen spinach

6 large eggs

¼ teaspoon salt

¼ teaspoon freshly ground black pepper

½ tablespoon coconut oil

½ large white onion, chopped

Preheat the oven to 350°F. Defrost the spinach in the microwave and drain well, or soak a bag in warm water until defrosted.

In a large bowl, whisk the eggs together and add the salt and pepper. Set aside.

In a pan, heat the coconut oil and sauté the onion until translucent, 3 to 5 minutes. Remove from the heat. Add the onion and spinach to the eggs and mix well.

Spoon the mixture into a twelve-compartment nonstick or greased muffin tin and bake for 15 to 20 minutes, or until the eggs are cooked through.

Western Egg Muffins

FOOD GROUP(S): N/A
MEAL PLAN: 3-DAY

---

208 calories, 3.6 g carbohydrates, 15.1 g fat, 4.5 g saturated fat,
14.3 g protein, 0.9 g fiber, 516.7 mg sodium per serving

The best part of these muffins is that they are basically foolproof. Follow the recipe as written or add whatever vegetables you have left over. These should be called Kitchen Sink Muffins! **SERVES 6 (2 MUFFINS PER SERVING)**

  1 tablespoon olive oil
  ½ onion, cut into small dice
  1 bell pepper, seeded and cut into small dice
  8 button mushrooms, quartered
  2 ounces spinach, washed well
  4 ounces bacon, cooked and diced
  6 large eggs

Preheat the oven to 325°F.

Heat the olive oil in a sauté pan. Add the onion and sauté until translucent. Add the bell pepper, sautéing until soft, then the mushrooms, sautéing briefly. Lastly, add the spinach and bacon and sauté for about 2 minutes. Remove from the heat.

Let the mixture cool for 5 minutes, then slowly whisk in eggs. Spoon the mixture into a nonstick or greased twelve-compartment muffin tin and bake until puffy and set.

Frittata

287.3 calories, 5.4 g carbohydrates, 20 g fat, 8.2 g saturated fat,
20.8 g protein, 1 g fiber, 802 mg sodium per serving

This frittata blew both of us away the first time we tried it—so delicious, so satisfying, and so easy to make. It's like a breakfast pizza, only healthier. **SERVES 4**

1 tablespoon coconut oil
½ onion, cut into small dice
2 cloves garlic, minced
½ pint cherry tomatoes
10 fresh basil leaves, cut into thin strips
1 teaspoon salt
1 teaspoon freshly ground black pepper
12 large eggs
4 ounces fresh mozzarella cheese, sliced thinly

Preheat the broiler.

Heat the coconut oil in an 12-inch ovenproof skillet and sauté the onion until translucent. Add the garlic and sauté for 2 minutes. Add the tomatoes and cook for 2 minutes, or until they just begin to pop. Next, add the basil, salt, pepper, and eggs and continue to cook over medium heat. When the edges are beginning to set, lift them with a spatula and roll the pan slightly so that uncooked egg can flow underneath and cook. When the eggs are about 75 percent set, 4 to 5 minutes or until egg mixture has set on the bottom and begins to set up on top add the mozzarella and broil in the oven until the top is set and the mozzarella is melted. Flip out of the pan onto a platter and serve immediately.

Soft-Boiled Eggs with Vegetables and Mustard Vinaigrette

FOOD GROUP(S): N/A
MEAL PLAN: 3-DAY

565 calories, 12.3 g carbohydrates, 51.5 g fat, 9.1 g saturated fat, 16.1 g protein, 3.6 g fiber, 691.7 mg sodium per serving

Nothing beats a runny egg over vegetables. It feels so indulgent, but you're getting so many nutrients, protein and fiber. This is also a great easy dinner! **SERVES 4**

2 red bell peppers
8 large eggs
¼ cup of chives, cut into ½-inch lengths
12 ounces spinach, washed well

Mustard Vinaigrette
2 tablespoons Dijon mustard
¼ cup balsamic vinegar
¾ cup extra-virgin olive oil
1 tablespoon fresh rosemary, chopped
½ tablespoon tarragon, chopped
1 tablespoon sage, chopped
½ teaspoon salt
½ teaspoon freshly ground black pepper

Preheat the broiler. Arrange the peppers on a baking sheet and place on the top rack in the oven. Watch closely and turn the peppers around with tongs as they begin to get splotchy. Continue to turn the peppers until each entire pepper has been darkened. Place the peppers in a bowl (be careful; they will be very hot) and cover the bowl with plastic wrap. Wait 15 to 20 minutes, until the peppers are cool enough to handle, and pull the stem out of each pepper. Hold one end of the pepper down on a flat surface and gently peel off the skin—this should happen easily. Cut open the pepper, scrape out and discard the seeds, and slice thinly.

Fill a medium-size pot with water and bring to a boil. Turn the heat down to a simmer. Add the eggs still in the shell and simmer for 5 to 7 minutes.

Prepare the vinaigrette: While the eggs are in the pot, place all ingredients for the vinaigrette in a small bowl or cup and whisk well. In a large bowl, toss the pepper, vinaigrette, and spinach together. Divide among four individual plates.

When the eggs are done, take out of the pot and carefully peel off their shells. Place two poached eggs on top of each salad and serve.

Overnight Oats

FOOD GROUP(S): 1 DAIRY, 1 STARCH
MEAL PLAN: WEEK 3

146.5 calories, 18.2 g carbohydrates, 3 g fat, 0.4 g saturated fat, 11.5 g protein, 3.6 g fiber, 36.5 mg sodium per serving

This is a whole new take on oatmeal. Prepare the night before and in the morning you have an amazing oatmeal ready for you right in your fridge. Add a spoonful of peanut or almond butter before you eat, to make it even more decadent. **SERVES 2**

½ cup old-fashioned rolled oats
⅔ cup unsweetened almond, coconut, or regular milk
½ cup plain Greek yogurt
1 teaspoon vanilla extract
½ teaspoon ground cinnamon
¼ teaspoon ground ginger

Mix all the ingredients together and seal in an airtight container. Refrigerate overnight and enjoy in the morning.

FOOD GROUP(S): N/A
MEAL PLAN: 3-DAY

Tofu Scramble

132 calories, 7.3 g carbohydrates, 8.2 g fat, 2.9 g saturated fat,
10 g protein, 2.2 g fiber, 320.8 mg sodium per serving

The turmeric in this scramble turns plain old tofu into a delicious golden yellow that could fool any egg lover. Loaded with vegetables, this vegetarian breakfast is quick and filling. **SERVES 4**

- 1 tablespoon coconut oil
- 2 cloves garlic, minced
- 1 medium-size yellow or white onion, diced finely
- 1 bell pepper, seeded and chopped
- 1 (14-ounce) package extra-firm tofu, drained and chopped into ½-inch cubes
- ½ teaspoon ground turmeric
- ¼ teaspoon chili powder
- ½ teaspoon salt
- 2 cups baby spinach, washed well

Heat a large pan over medium-high heat and add the coconut oil. Add the garlic and heat until aromatic. Add the onion and sauté for 1 minute, then add the pepper. Sauté until the pepper is tender and the onion is translucent, stirring occasionally, about 5 minutes. Next, add the tofu, stirring to incorporate, then stir in the spices and salt until the tofu turns bright yellow. Lastly, add the spinach and cook covered for 1 to 2 minutes, until wilted. Serve immediately.

Appetizers

Edamame Salad

FOOD GROUP(S): N/A
MEAL PLAN: WEEK 1

139.3 calories, 11.9 g carbohydrates, 6.3 g fat, 0.5 g saturated fat,
7.9 g protein, 4.9 g fiber, 340 mg sodium per serving

A perfect side dish on a hot day! This edamame salad is packed with protein and fiber without tasting bland. The rice vinegar dressing gives it a fresh taste that will only be better for leftovers. **SERVES 4**

   1 (10-ounce) package frozen, shelled edamame, thawed
   1 cup shredded carrots (about 2 medium-size)
   ½ teaspoon salt
   ½ teaspoon freshly ground black pepper
   1 tablespoon sesame oil
   1½ tablespoons rice vinegar
   2 scallions, chopped
   ¼ cup chopped fresh cilantro

Place all the ingredients in a large mixing bowl. Mix well and let sit for 15 to 20 minutes in the refrigerator before serving to really bring out the flavors.

Shepherd's Salad

FOOD GROUP(S): N/A
MEAL PLAN: WEEK 1

58 calories, 6.4 g carbohydrates, 3.8 g fat, 0.5 g saturated fat,
1.3 g protein, 1.8 g fiber, 587 mg sodium per serving

Sometimes the simplest foods are the best. This crunchy and tangy salad is beautiful to look at and so easy to make. Turn it into an entrée salad by topping with some protein, such as grilled tofu, fish or chicken. **SERVES 4**

1 pint cherry tomatoes, halved

1 bell pepper, seeded and cut into small dice

1 medium-size cucumber, cut into small dice

1 clove garlic, minced

1 tablespoon extra-virgin olive oil

1 teaspoon salt

1 teaspoon freshly ground black pepper

2 tablespoons freshly squeezed lemon juice

Place all the ingredients in a large mixing bowl. Mix well and let sit for at least 5 to 10 minutes to soak up the flavors.

Spinach Hummus

FOOD GROUP(S): N/A
MEAL PLAN: 3-DAY

59 calories, 6.4 g carbohydrates, 2.8 g fat, 0.3 g saturated fat, 2.5 g protein, 1.5 g fiber, 123.7 mg sodium per serving

Hummus is a great vehicle to flavor up. This spinach hummus makes a great snack or appetizer, as it's packed with protein and fiber! It's especially great with chopped veggies or fiber crackers (Week 1). **SERVES 20 (2 TABLESPOONS PER SERVING)**

2 cups chickpeas (If using canned, drain and rinse.)

1 cup spinach, packed, washed well

¼ cup freshly squeezed lemon juice

3 cloves garlic

1½ tablespoons tahini

2 tablespoons extra-virgin olive oil

1 teaspoon salt

1 teaspoon freshly ground black pepper

Place all the ingredients in the bowl of a food processor and puree until smooth. Refrigerate, and serve chilled.

Steamed Artichokes with Lemon Dipping Sauce

FOOD GROUP(S): N/A
MEAL PLAN: 3-DAY

388 calories, 19.6 g carbohydrates, 2.2 g fat, 0 g saturated fat, 4.5 g protein, 7.4 g fiber, 366.8 mg sodium

Artichokes are always a great appetizer or snack. They take awhile to eat and keep your hands busy. They're filled with fiber and antioxidants, and when dipped in the tangy lemon sauce, are beyond delicious. **SERVES 4**

4 medium-size artichokes
1 lemon, cut in half

Lemon Dipping Sauce
½ cup low-fat mayonnaise
3 cloves garlic, minced
2 teaspoons freshly squeezed lemon juice
1 teaspoon lemon zest

Cut off the artichoke stems so they can sit flat. Using kitchen scissors, trim off the pointy parts of all the leaves. Take the lemon halves and rub all over the artichokes, squeezing the excess juice into each artichoke center. Fill a large saucepan with 2 to 3 inches of water. Slice the lemon halves and place in the saucepan. Place the artichokes in steamer rack, set the rack in the saucepan, cover, and steam for about 40 minutes, or until the leaves pull out easily. Remove from the heat and allow to drain and cool. Open the artichokes and scoop out the inedible choke and purple-toned small inner leaves, using a small spoon or ice-cream scooper.

Place all the dipping sauce ingredients in a small bowl and whisk well. Use as a dip for the leaves.

FOOD GROUP(S): N/A
MEAL PLAN: 3-DAY

Ceviche

82.5 calories, 5.7 g carbohydrates, 5.3 g fat, 0.9 g saturated fat,
16.2 g protein, 0.9 g fiber, 353.8 mg sodium per serving

Who says fish has to be boring? Ceviche, especially popular in Central and South America, is "cooked" with the acids from the lime juice. Its bold flavors make it a great treat on hot day! **SERVES 4**

- 12 ounces white fish (e.g., sea bass or red snapper), cut into
  ¼ inch dice
- ⅔ cup freshly squeezed lime juice
- 1½ tablespoons finely diced serrano chile
- 2 tablespoons finely diced yellow bell pepper
- 2 tablespoons finely diced red bell pepper
- 2 tablespoons minced red onion
- 1 teaspoon minced garlic
- 2 tablespoons chopped fresh cilantro
- 1 tablespoon extra-virgin olive oil
- ½ teaspoon salt
- 1 lime, sliced for garnish

Place the fish, lime juice, serrano chile, yellow and red bell pepper, red onion, garlic, and cilantro in a large bowl. Mix well to cover every surface of the fish, cover, and refrigerate for 3 to 4 hours. Toss with the cilantro, olive oil, and salt, and divide among four plates. Garnish with lime and serve.

FOOD GROUP(S): N/A
MEAL PLAN: WEEK 1

Summer Rolls

80.2 calories, 6.9 g carbohydrates, 4 g fat, 0.6 g saturated fat,
6.3 g protein, 2.4 g fiber, 204.4 mg sodium per serving

Bored with salad? Well roll your veggies up with some tofu and a great dipping sauce, and *voilà!* no fork required. **MAKES 10 ROLLS, OR ABOUT 3 SERVINGS**

Filling

2 cups bean sprouts

2 carrots, julienned

1 tablespoon sesame oil

3 tablespoons chopped fresh cilantro

1 bell pepper, seeded and julienned

10 ounces firm tofu, sliced into ½-inch-thick strips

Juice of 1 lime

10 Bibb lettuce leaves

Dipping Sauce

Juice of 2 limes

2 tablespoons soy sauce

2 teaspoons minced jalapeño pepper

1 teaspoon minced garlic

1 teaspoon red pepper flakes

In a large bowl, stir together all the filling ingredients except the lettuce. Lay 1 piece of lettuce down on a cutting board. Spoon ¼ cup of filling into the lettuce and fold the left and right sides over like a burrito. Continue with all the other lettuce leafs.

Mix dipping sauce ingredients and use for dipping.

Grilled Zucchini with Sage Goat Cheese Filling

FOOD GROUP(S): 1/2 DAIRY
MEAL PLAN: WEEK 1

89.3 calories, 4.7 g carbohydrates, 7 g fat, 2.8 g saturated fat, 3.6 g protein, 1.2 g fiber, 644.5 mg sodium per serving

Grilled vegetables take on such depth of flavors. Adding the goat cheese and sage takes a simple vegetable to a whole new dimension. We love serving these at dinner parties. **SERVES: 4**

2 zucchini, cut lengthwise into ¼-inch-thick slices

1 tablespoon extra-virgin olive oil

½ teaspoon salt

½ teaspoon freshly ground black pepper
1½ ounces goat cheese
1 tablespoon chopped fresh parsley
½ teaspoon freshly squeezed lemon juice
1 teaspoon chopped fresh sage
⅓ cup fresh basil leaves, chopped
1 tablespoon balsamic vinegar

Preheat the grill. Brush the zucchini strips with the olive oil, and season with the salt and pepper. Grill for 4 minutes per side.

While the zucchini cooks, blend together the goat cheese, parsley, lemon juice, and sage in a bowl.

Lay out the zucchini strips and spread the goat cheese mixture thinly onto each. Top with the basil leaves. Roll up and serve, drizzled with balsamic vinegar.

Broccoli and Mushroom Soup

FOOD GROUP(S): N/A
MEAL PLAN: 3-DAY

86.7 calories, 13.6 g carbohydrates, 3 g fat, 0.4 g saturated fat,
5.5 g protein, 4.5 g fiber, 52.7 mg sodium per serving

Mushrooms bring a texture and flavor profile to this soup that makes it so satisfying. The earthiness of the mushrooms and broccoli complement so well with the brightness of the parsley and lemon juice. It's a perfectly balanced soup for any kind of weather! SERVES 6

1 tablespoon extra-virgin olive oil
1 medium-size onion, diced
2 cloves garlic, minced
1 teaspoon red pepper flakes
2 pounds broccoli, florets only
2 teaspoons freshly squeezed lemon juice
6 ounces button mushrooms, chopped
2 tablespoons parsley

Heat the olive oil in a pot. Add the onion and sauté until soft. Add the garlic and pepper flakes and sauté for 1 minute. Add the broccoli and sauté for 3 to 5 minutes. Add the lemon juice and 1/2 cup of water and cover. Steam for 5 minutes, until the broccoli is almost done. Add the mushrooms and sauté briefly. Puree with an immersion blender and serve. Garnish with the parsley.

Raw Oysters

FOOD GROUP(S): N/A
MEAL PLAN: 3-DAY

166 calories, 11.2 g carbohydrates, 4.6 g fat, 1 g saturated fat, 19 g protein, 0.2 g fiber, 212 mg sodium per serving

Raw oysters are not just for romantic date nights. Ask your fishmonger to shuck them for you; transport them with ice; and you'll have a very simple, easy, yet very sophisticated appetizer in no time! **SERVES 4**

1 tablespoon minced fresh sage
½ teaspoon minced fresh tarragon
Zest and juice of 1 lemon
16 fresh oysters, shucked

In a small bowl or cup, stir together the herbs and lemon zest. Lay out the oysters on a platter or individual plates. Place some of the herb mixture and lemon juice on each. Serve immediately.

Black Bean Salad

FOOD GROUP(S): N/A
MEAL PLAN: WEEK 1

210.5 calories, 25 g carbohydrates, 10.1 g fat, 1.3 g saturated fat, 7.7 g protein, 9.9 g fiber, 260.5 mg sodium per serving

Not just for vegetarians, this black bean salad is almost creamy, thanks to the avocado. Like it hot? Then add more jalapeño—or leave it out, if you prefer a mild version. We love it with extra lime juice, for a tart boost. **SERVES 4**

1 (15-ounce) can black beans, drained and rinsed

2 medium-size tomatoes, chopped

½ medium-size red onion, chopped

½ bunch scallions, chopped

1 jalapeño pepper, seeded

1 avocado, peeled, pitted, and diced

¼ teaspoon salt, or more to taste

¼ teaspoon freshly ground black pepper

Zest and juice of 1 lime

½ tablespoon extra-virgin olive oil

1 tablespoon red wine vinegar

1 bunch fresh cilantro, chopped

In a large bowl, toss together all the ingredients except the cilantro, top with the cilantro, and serve.

Entrées

Baked Chicken with Asparagus and Mushroom Salad

FOOD GROUP(S): N/A
MEAL PLAN: WEEK 2 (if you use Sugar Detox Vinaigrette [page 178], it's good for the 3-Day)

458.5 calories, 25.5 g carbohydrates, 24 g fat, 2.6 g saturated fat, 37.2 g protein, 7.5 g fiber, 1358.8 mg sodium per serving

We tested this recipe together with four other people and the results were unanimous. We all flipped over this chicken and salad dish. With typical "meat and potatoes" guys at the table with us who were gladly finishing each bite, we knew we had a winner here! SERVES 4

Baked Chicken
4 tablespoons chopped fresh cilantro
3 cloves garlic, minced
1 tablespoon olive oil
Juice of ½ lemon
1 teaspoon salt
1 teaspoon freshly ground black pepper
4 whole chicken breasts

Asparagus and Mushroom Salad
1 pound asparagus, base trimmed
2 tablespoons extra-virgin olive oil
½ teaspoon salt
½ teaspoon freshly ground black pepper
1 pound sliced mushrooms (e.g., cremini, shiitake)
1 pound spinach, washed well
Lemon wedges

Fresh Raspberry Dressing
¼ cup almond oil

¼ cup fresh raspberries, mashed with a fork

½ teaspoon chopped fresh rosemary

¾ cup champagne vinegar

½ teaspoons salt

½ teaspoons freshly ground black pepper

Place the cilantro, garlic, olive oil, lemon juice, salt, and pepper in a large bowl and mix well. Place the chicken in this mixture, cover, and refrigerate for 1 hour. At the half-hour point, preheat the oven to 375°F. Remove the chicken from its marinade, place in a single layer in a baking pan, and bake for 18 to 22 minutes, or until done. Discard the remaining marinade.

While the chicken is baking, prepare the salad: Toss the asparagus in 1 tablespoon of the olive oil and half of each of the salt and pepper, place in a separate baking pan, and roast for 8 to 10 minutes or until tender. Do the same for the mushrooms, separately, using the remaining tablespoon of olive oil and remaining salt and pepper.

Prepare the dressing: Place all the ingredients for the salad dressing in a small bowl and whisk together well. When chicken is done, toss the spinach in the salad dressing to coat. Divide the spinach among four plates. Split up the vegetables evenly among the four plates. Add the chicken and serve with lemon wedges.

Salsa Verde Chicken

FOOD GROUP(S): N/A
MEAL PLAN: 3-DAY

320.3 calories, 12.5 g carbohydrates, 22.6 g fat, 7.8 g saturated fat, 18.3 g protein, 4.3 g fiber, 658.3 mg sodium per serving

Tomatillos, also called *tomate verde* in Mexico for their green color, are a staple in Mexican cooking. Broiling them yields a great smoky flavor for the entire dish. Cooking the chicken thighs on the bone keeps the chicken moist and delicious, and the avocado adds a final touch of creamy texture. **SERVES 4**

1 pound tomatillos, husked

1 serrano chile or 2 jalapeño peppers, stemmed and seeded

4 chicken thighs, bone-in, skin on

1 tablespoon coconut oil (vegetable oil may be used)

1 medium-size onion, diced

3 cloves garlic, minced

½ cup roughly chopped fresh cilantro

1 teaspoon salt, or to taste

½ avocado, peeled, pitted, and diced

Preheat the broiler.

Place the tomatillos and chile on a baking sheet. Broil for about 5 minutes on each side, until the tomatillos start to blister and soften. Remove from the oven and set aside, then place chicken thighs, skin side up, on the same baking sheet and broil until the chicken browns, 10 to 12 minutes.

While the chicken is cooking, heat the coconut oil in a saucepan over medium heat. Add the onion and garlic and cook, stirring occasionally, until they soften, about 5 minutes. Turn off the heat, add tomatillos and chile to the same pot, and use an immersion blender to blend everything together. Turn the heat back on to medium-low and bring the sauce to a simmer. Add the chicken thighs to the sauce, cover, and cook until the chicken is cooked through, about 25 minutes. Add the cilantro and salt before serving. Top with the diced avocado.

Serving suggestion: Spoon the chicken and sauce over steamed spinach or other leafy greens. The chicken may be served with 1/2 cup of cooked brown rice or a whole wheat tortilla (see approved-brands, page 233) during or after Week 4.

Zucchini "Pasta"

FOOD GROUP(S): N/A
MEAL PLAN: 3-DAY

124 calories, 8.4 g carbohydrates, 9 g fat, 7 g saturated fat,
5.3 g protein, 2.5 g fiber, 409.3 mg sodium per serving

Pasta cravings get satisfied with this play on noodles here. Make extra and serve them cold the next day with some extra lemon squeezed on top. **SERVES 4**

  2 pounds zucchini
  2 tablespoons coconut oil
  2 cloves garlic, minced
  ½ teaspoon salt

Wash and dry the zucchini. Cut off the bottom and top stems. Using a vegetable peeler, peel a zucchini into lengthwise "noodles," peeling off several ribbons from one side and then on another side once you hit the seeded core. Continue to do this around the zucchini until the core is left, then discard the core. Repeat with remaining zucchini.

In a pan, heat 1 tablespoon of the coconut oil and sauté half of the garlic. Add half of zucchini and sauté until it softens and begins to turn translucent. Remove from the heat. Cook the remaining zucchini with the remaining oil and garlic. Place the zucchini in a large bowl, sprinkle with salt, and toss. Serve immediately.

Poached Chicken Breasts

FOOD GROUP(S): N/A
MEAL PLAN: 3-DAY

303.8 calories, 11.1 g carbohydrates, 5.1 g fat, 1.3 g saturated fat,
45.6 g protein, 1.5 g fiber, 747 mg sodium per serving

Chicken doesn't have to be boring—it just takes a little finesse to make it mouthwatering. Poaching the chicken keeps it nice and tender while infusing a great flavor. Serve with Zucchini "Pasta" (above).
SERVES 4

1½ pounds boneless, skinless chicken breast

½ teaspoon salt

½ teaspoon freshly ground black pepper

1 quart chicken stock

½ cup white wine

1 sprig fresh rosemary

2 sprigs fresh parsley

2 sprigs fresh thyme

8 peppercorns

8 coriander seeds

1 lemon, cut in half

Sprinkle chicken with the salt and pepper. Set aside.

Combine the chicken stock, white wine, rosemary, parsley, thyme, peppercorns, and coriander in a medium-size saucepan. Squeeze the lemon halves into the mixture and toss the squeezed halves into the liquid. Bring to a boil and lower the heat to a simmer. Simmer for 30 minutes. Strain out the spices and lemon halves.

Add the chicken to the broth and bring it back to a simmer. Cook covered for 15 to 18 minutes, or until the chicken is cooked through.

Herb-Roasted Chicken

FOOD GROUP(S): N/A
MEAL PLAN: 3-DAY

277.4 calories, 5.6 g carbohydrates, 4.1 g fat, 1.5 g saturated fat, 44.2 g protein, 0.7 g fiber, 444.1 mg sodium per serving

Nothing is better than a roasted chicken, in our opinion. This one especially is so flavorful and moist, thanks to the lemon being cooked inside the chicken. All the herbs and spices are a great counterbalance to the roasting effect and leftovers are perfect on top of a simple salad. **SERVES 4**

1 (3- to 5-pound) whole chicken

1 tablespoon finely chopped fresh rosemary

1 teaspoon dried marjoram

1 teaspoon dried sage

¼ teaspoon cayenne

½ teaspoon salt

½ teaspoon freshly ground black pepper

1 tablespoon freshly squeezed lemon juice

1 tablespoon olive oil

1 lemon, cut in half

Rinse the chicken and pat dry with paper towels, then place in a baking dish.

In a small bowl, mix together the rosemary, marjoram, sage, cayenne, salt, black pepper, lemon juice, and olive oil. Rub the marinade all over the chicken. Take the two lemon halves and place them inside chicken cavity. Cover and let marinate for at least 2 hours in the refrigerator.

Preheat the oven to 425°F. Place the chicken in the oven (discard the marinade) and immediately lower the temperature to 375°F. Roast for about 1 1/2 hours, or until the chicken is thoroughly cooked through. If the chicken skin starts to burn before the rest of the bird is ready, cover with foil.

Chicken Fajitas

FOOD GROUP(S): 1 STARCH
MEAL PLAN: WEEK 4
(Can be eaten as early as 3-Day, if no tortilla.)

302.5 calories, 30 g carbohydrates, 11.6 g fat, 5.9 g saturated fat, 34.6 g protein, 13.6 g fiber, 965 mg sodium per serving

Always a crowd-pleaser, fajitas can be done well or turn into a Sugar Detox disaster. These fajitas have just the right mix of spice and flavors. Opt for tofu here if you're a vegetarian or to just mix it up. If you're still in the early weeks and aren't allowed to have tortillas yet, use lettuce as wraps or simply eat this dish on a plate. **SERVES 4**

½ cup chopped fresh cilantro

2 cloves garlic, minced

2 tablespoons freshly squeezed lime juice
2 tablespoons low sodium soy sauce
½ teaspoon chili powder
¼ teaspoon salt
1 pound boneless, skinless chicken breast, sliced into 1–inch strips
2 tablespoons coconut oil
1 onion, sliced
1 red bell pepper, seeded and sliced
1 yellow bell pepper, seeded and sliced
4 tortillas (see approved brands, page 233)

In a bowl large enough to hold the chicken, combine the cilantro, garlic, lime juice, soy sauce, chili powder, salt, and 1/4 cup of water and mix well. Add the chicken and make sure it is well coated. Cover and place in refrigerator for at least an hour.

In a large saucepan, heat the coconut oil. Add the chicken (discard the marinade) and cook for 4 minutes. Add the onion and peppers and sauté until the chicken and vegetables are cooked through, 3 to 5 minutes. Remove from the heat and set aside.

Turn on your stove top and using tongs, place the tortillas directly on top of the flame for 10 seconds each side, carefully making sure that they don't burn. Divide the chicken and vegetables among the tortillas.

Turkey Meatballs in Marinara Sauce

FOOD GROUP(S): N/A
MEAL PLAN: WEEK 1

509.3 calories, 12.2 g carbohydrates, 28.5 g fat, 11.1 g saturated fat, 49.3 g protein, 2.9 g fiber, 452.5 mg sodium per serving

Comfort food takes on a healthy twist here. These meatballs are light and delicious and the homemade marinara sauce is far superior to anything you can find in a jar. Try serving the meatballs over sautéed spinach to complete the meal. Although there is Parmesan cheese in the recipe, 1/2 cup goes a long way and is small enough that it won't count toward your dairy servings. Just don't make these during the 3-Day Fix, and you're good to go! SERVES 4 (MAKES ABOUT 16 MEATBALLS)

Marinara Sauce
1 tablespoon coconut oil
1 large onion, chopped
2 cloves garlic, minced
1 tablespoon dried oregano
¾ pound tomatoes, chopped

Turkey Meatballs
2 pounds ground turkey
1 medium-size onion, chopped in small pieces
½ stalk celery, chopped small
¼ cup chopped fresh parsley
1 tablespoon chopped fresh sage
2 large eggs
½ cup Parmesan cheese
1 tablespoon chopped fresh rosemary

Preheat the oven to 350°F.

Prepare the sauce: In a large saucepan, heat the oil over medium-high heat and sauté the onion until translucent. Add the garlic and oregano and sauté for 1 minute. Add the chopped tomatoes and cook down for 10 to 15 minutes.

While the sauce is cooking, place all the meatball ingredients in a large bowl and mix well. Using an ice-cream scooper, make 1 1/2-inch-meatballs. Place the meatballs on a baking sheet and bake for 12 to 15 minutes.

Add the meatballs to the sauce and simmer for 15 to 20 minutes, or until meatballs are completely cooked through.

Turkey Sliders

FOOD GROUP(S): 1 STARCH
MEAL PLAN: WEEK 4

628.5 calories, 46.9 g carbohydrates, 29.6 g fat, 9.7 g saturated fat, 44.9 g protein, 0 g fiber, 491 mg sodium per serving

This recipe from Chef Charis West has a cool twist of adding apple as a way to prevent these sliders from turning into hockey pucks and keep them nice and moist. If you're in Week 1, 2, or 3, use lettuce wraps or put the burgers on top of a salad. **SERVES 2**

1 Granny Smith apple
1 tablespoon Dijon mustard
½ cup chopped chives or green onions
12 ounces ground turkey
Salt
Freshly ground black pepper
½ avocado, peeled, pitted, and sliced
1 to 2 ounces sliced provolone
Approved bread product for buns (see page 233) or lettuce

Peel and grate the apple with a cheese grater and squeeze out a bit of the juice, but do not squeeze it completely dry. Add the grated apple, chives, mustard, salt, and pepper to the turkey and form into four small patties. Cook the burgers in a skillet over medium-high heat for 4 to 5 minutes each side until cooked through. Serve topped with the cheese and avocado slices.

Cajun Dirty Brown Rice

FOOD GROUP(S): 1 STARCH
MEAL PLAN: WEEK 4

322 calories, 40.3 g carbohydrates, 8.7 g fat, 2.2 g saturated fat, 20.7 g protein, 3.3 g fiber, 151.3 mg sodium per serving

This is a healthy version of the Louisiana favorite, dirty rice, from Chef Charis West. Generally, it is richly flavored with chicken liver or giblets, which have been replaced by ground turkey and mushrooms.

The texture and flavor resemble the traditional recipe, but don't be fooled . . . this ain't your momma's dirty rice! Vegetarians can substitute beans for the turkey to make this a meatless option. **SERVES 4**

1 cup uncooked brown rice
8 ounces cremini or button mushrooms, chopped finely
1 pound ground turkey
2 stalks celery, chopped finely
½ green bell pepper, chopped finely
3 green onions, chopped finely
¼ cup finely chopped fresh parsley
Creole seasoning, preferably Tony Chachere's brand

In a saucepan, bring 2½ cups of water to a boil, then add the rice. Lower the heat to low and simmer covered for about 40 minutes, or until all the water has been absorbed.

While the rice is cooking, brown the mushrooms and turkey in a large skillet until cooked through. Remove the turkey mixture and sauté the celery and green bell pepper until cooked through, about 7 minutes. Return the turkey mixture to the skillet and stir in the cooked rice, green onions, and parsley. Season to taste with liberal amounts of Creole seasoning.

Summer Shrimp Pasta Salad

FOOD GROUP(S): 1 STARCH
MEAL PLAN: WEEK 3

294.3 calories, 18.3 g carbohydrates, 8.6 g fat, 1.3 g saturated fat, 37.6 g protein, 4.3 g fiber, 177.4 mg sodium per serving

This shrimp pasta salad has been a family favorite for years. As soon as the weather starts getting warm again, the requests for this dish start coming. Shrimp takes the main stage, with the whole wheat pasta as supporting role, in this room-temperature entrée. I often triple the recipe for a big barbecue and there is rarely anything left over. **SERVES 4**

1 cup uncooked whole wheat rotini (approved brand; see page 237)
1½ pounds large shrimp, peeled and deveined

½ pint cherry tomatoes, halved

¾ cup sliced celery

½ cup peeled, pitted, and chopped avocado

½ cup seeded and chopped poblano chile

2 tablespoons chopped fresh cilantro

2 teaspoons grated lemon zest

3 tablespoons freshly squeezed lemon juice

2 teaspoons extra-virgin olive oil

¾ teaspoon kosher salt

Bring 8 cups water to a boil in a large saucepan. Add the pasta to the pan and cook for 5 minutes, or until almost tender. Add the shrimp to the pasta and cook for 3 minutes, or until done. Drain. Rinse with cold water and drain well. Combine the pasta mixture, tomatoes, celery, avocado, chile, cilantro, lemon zest and juice, olive oil, and salt in a large bowl; toss well.

Baked Shrimp with Spinach and Tomato

FOOD GROUP(S): N/A
MEAL PLAN: WEEK 1

353.5 calories, 17.4 g carbohydrates, 9.2 g fat, 4.9 g saturated fat, 50.5 g protein, 2.4 g fiber, 492.5 mg sodium per serving

This dish comes out steaming hot and warms the soul. The tomatoes turn into a great sauce for the spinach and the shrimp always end up extra tender! SERVES 2

2 teaspoons coconut oil

2 cloves garlic, minced

1 medium-size white onion, diced small

2 teaspoons fresh rosemary

⅛ teaspoon salt

Freshly ground black pepper

6 cups spinach, washed well

2 tomatoes, diced

1 pound shrimp, cleaned and deveined

Preheat the oven to 425°F.

In a large saucepan, heat the olive oil and add the garlic and onion, stirring until translucent. Add the rosemary and salt, and then add pepper to taste. Add the spinach and cook until wilted. Next, add the tomatoes and cook for 1 minute. Then add the shrimp, stir, and remove from the heat.

Transfer the shrimp mixture to an ovenproof dish and bake for 12 to 15, minutes or until the shrimp is pink and not translucent inside.

Crabmeat and Caper Salad

FOOD GROUP(S): N/A
MEAL PLAN: 3-DAY

220 calories, 20 g carbohydrates, 7.5 g fat, 1 g saturated fat,
22.7 g protein, 4.7 g fiber, 994.5 mg sodium per serving

This colorful crabmeat salad is a great way to get in those healthy omega-3 fatty acids. The saltiness of the capers pair so nicely with the sweetness of the peppers, and the crab shines with the lemon and vinegar. **SERVES 4**

1 pound jumbo lump crabmeat
⅓ cup seeded and chopped colorful bell peppers
2 bunches green onion, chopped
½ teaspoon garlic powder
Juice of 3 lemons
3 ounces seasoned rice wine vinegar
2 tablespoons extra-virgin olive oil
⅓ cup chopped celery
Sea salt
½ teaspoon cayenne
3 to 4 tablespoons capers
1 tablespoon chopped fresh cilantro (optional)
Endive leaves, for serving

In a bowl, fold all of the above, except the endive leaves, until well mixed. Cover and refrigerate for 3 to 4 hours before serving. Serve on top of the endive leaves.

Mustard-Crusted Salmon

FOOD GROUP(S): N/A
MEAL PLAN: 3-DAY

371.3 calories, 1 g carbohydrates, 23.7g fat, 4.5 g saturated fat,
34 g protein, 0 g fiber, 353.3 mg sodium per serving

This is a dish that seems super fancy but is incredibly simple to make. Normally, traditional versions of this recipe use bread crumbs to make the mustard topping a bit thicker, but we don't think you'll miss it at all. **SERVES 4**

4 (6-ounce) salmon fillets, skin removed
⅛ teaspoon salt
⅛ teaspoon freshly ground black pepper
2 cloves garlic
¾ teaspoon fresh rosemary
1½ tablespoons extra-virgin olive oil
2 tablespoons Dijon mustard
2 tablespoons whole-grain mustard

Preheat the broiler. Line a baking sheet with foil and place the salmon on the foil. Sprinkle the salmon with salt and pepper.

In a blender, whirl the garlic, rosemary, olive oil, and mustards until well mixed. Broil the salmon for 2 minutes, remove from the oven and spoon on the mustard sauce. Broil for an additional 5 minutes, or until cooked through.

Poached Halibut with Ginger-Lime Sauce

FOOD GROUP(S): N/A
MEAL PLAN: 3-DAY

261 calories, 2.2 g carbohydrates, 10.7 g fat, 1.5 g saturated fat,
36.7 g protein, 0.5 g fiber, 554.5 mg sodium per serving

This is another dish that seems so tricky but is so simple to make. Poaching the halibut is a great way to keep the integrity of the fish without adding any Sugar Detox concerns of AGEs. The sauce is so amazing, you might have to stop yourself from eating it by the spoon-ful! **SERVES 4**

  5 quarter-size slices peeled fresh ginger
  4 scallions, sliced
  4 (6-ounce) halibut fillets

Ginger-Lime Sauce
  2 tablespoons soy sauce
  2 tablespoons sesame oil
  1½ tablespoons freshly squeezed lime juice
  ¼ teaspoon ground ginger

Prepare the halibut: Fill a large saucepan with 1/2-inch layer of water. Add the ginger slices and scallions. Bring the water to a boil and lower the heat to a simmer. Add the halibut and cover. Simmer for 5 to 7 minutes, or until no longer translucent in the middle.

While the halibut cooks, place all sauce ingredients in a small bowl and mix.

Serve each piece of halibut with 1 tablespoon of sauce.

Fish Tacos with Roasted Peach Salsa

FOOD GROUP(S): 1 FRUIT
MEAL PLAN: WEEK 3

364.3 calories, 47.1 g carbohydrates, 11.4 g fat, 1.3 g saturated fat, 32.5 g protein, 16.6 g fiber, 742.8 mg sodium per serving

Roasted peaches add an unexpected twist to this otherwise simple fish taco recipe. **SERVES 4**

  1 pound white fish (e.g., cod, haddock), cut into strips
  2 tablespoons olive oil
  ½ teaspoon salt
  ½ teaspoon freshly ground black pepper
  Tortillas (approved brand; see page 233)
  Lemon slices

Roasted Peach Salsa

2 peaches, halved and pitted

4 Roma tomatoes

1 medium-size onion, quartered

1 jalapeño pepper

½ bunch fresh cilantro, chopped

Salt

Freshly ground black pepper

Preheat the oven to 400°F.

Prepare the fish: Cut the fish into ¼-by-¼–inch pieces. Toss in the olive oil, salt, and pepper, and roast until done and flakes easily, 5 to 8 minutes.

To prepare the salsa, preheat the oven to 350°F. Roast the peaches, tomatoes, onion, and jalapeño in a pan until caramelized. Remove the seeds from the jalapeño and place all the salsa ingredients in a blender, processing until smooth. Keep hot until needed.

Wrap the tortillas in a moist paper towel and microwave for 1 minute. After the tortillas are warmed and the fish is done, assemble the tacos. Top with the salsa and serve with the lemon slices.

Miso-Glazed White Fish with Vegetables

FOOD GROUP(S): N/A
MEAL PLAN: WEEK 2

379.5 calories, 22.3 g carbohydrates, 16.9 g fat, 2.5 g saturated fat, 36 g protein, 6.6 g fiber, 636 mg sodium per serving

---

Miso, a Japanese seasoning that's produced by fermenting rice, barley, and soybeans, adds an amazing complexity to plain old white fish, making this dish a delicious addition to any meal plan. **SERVES 4**

¼ cup white miso

4 tablespoons sesame oil

2 tablespoons mirin

4 (6-ounce) pieces white fish (e.g., cod or halibut)

1 onion, sliced

1 carrot, julienned

1 head broccoli, florets only

1 tablespoon sesame seeds, toasted

1 cup fresh string beans

1 tablespoon chopped fresh cilantro, for garnish

Preheat the oven to 375°F. Place the miso, 1 teaspoon of the sesame oil, and the mirin in a small bowl and mix. Place the fish in a baking dish and cover with the mixture.

Heat the remaining ounce of sesame oil in the pan and sauté the onion quickly, 3 to 5 minutes. Add the carrot and sauté for 2 minutes. Add the broccoli and ¼ cup of water and cover. Steam until done, 8 to 10 minutes.

While broccoli is steaming, put the fish in the oven and bake for 10 to 12 minutes. Add the string beans to vegetables for the last minute of cooking. Plate and garnish with the cilantro.

Braised Short Ribs

FOOD GROUP(S): N/A
MEAL PLAN: WEEK 2

284.5 calories, 35 g carbohydrates, 4.4 g fat, 0.7 g saturated fat,
5.6 g protein, 7.3 g fiber, 723 mg sodium to serve

These tender short ribs basically fall off the bone and melt in your mouth. Fortunately, the recipe only calls for just over half a bottle of wine, which means there is the perfect pairing left for the cook and his or her lucky guests! **SERVES 4**

1 tablespoon extra-virgin olive oil

4 bone-in short ribs

1 large onion, diced

1 tablespoon fresh rosemary

2 tablespoons fresh thyme

2 bay leaves

2 stalks celery, diced

2 carrots, diced

2 cloves garlic, chopped

1½ cups tomato paste

2 to 3 cups red wine

1 teaspoon salt

1 teaspoon freshly ground black pepper

Preheat the oven to 350°F.

Pour the olive oil into a Dutch oven and heat on the stovetop. Pat the ribs dry with paper towels and brown evenly on all four sides. Remove from the pan. Add the onion, rosemary, thyme, and bay leaves to the pan and sauté until tender. Add the celery and sauté for 2 to 3 minutes. Add the carrots and sauté for 4 to 5 minutes. Add the garlic and cook for 1 minute. Add the tomato paste and cook until browned. Add ½ cup of water and the wine. Place the ribs in veggie mixture.

Braise covered for 2 to 3 hours, checking every 30 minutes. Flip the ribs halfway through the cooking time and sprinkle with salt and pepper. After the ribs are cooked, remove 2 cups of the sauce, puree, and spoon over the ribs to serve.

Side Dishes

FOOD GROUP(S): N/A
MEAL PLAN: 3-DAY

Haricots Verts with Mint

70.3 calories, 12.8 g carbohydrates, 0.6 g fat, 0 g saturated fat,
2.3 g protein, 3.9 g fiber, 152.8 mg sodium per serving

Mint is an unexpected companion to these green beans but add a wonderful lightness to a great, simple side dish. **SERVES 4**

- 1 tablespoon olive oil
- 1 shallot, sliced
- 1 pound string beans
- ⅛ cup thinly sliced mint leaves
- ¼ teaspoon salt
- ¼ teaspoon freshly ground black pepper

Heat the olive oil in a saucepan, add the shallot, and sauté until tender. Add the string beans, sauté briefly, add 1/4 cup of water, and cover. Steam for 5 minutes. Remove from the heat, add the mint leaves, salt, and pepper, toss, and serve.

FOOD GROUP(S): N/A
MEAL PLAN: WEEK 1, WEEK 4 IF EATEN WITH PASTA

Pistachio Pesto

218.9 calories, 4.7 g carbohydrates, 21.5 g fat, 3.4 g saturated fat,
4.5 g protein, 1.7 g fiber, 193.3 mg sodium per serving

Using pistachios in this pesto is a great way to add more fiber and protein to a sauce. Use it for more than just pasta: Spread it on chicken, dip in veggies, or even mix with Zucchini "Pasta" (page 197). As this is a big portion, you can freeze the pesto and save for later.
SERVES 8 (2 TABLESPOONS PESTO PER SERVING)

½ cup fresh basil, packed

1 cup shelled unsalted pistachios

2 cloves garlic

¼ cup grated Parmesan cheese

½ teaspoon salt

¼ to ½ cup extra-virgin olive oil

Place the basil, pistachios, garlic, Parmesan, and salt in a blender. Process until well blended. Beginning with 1/4 cup of the olive oil, add the oil slowly while the blender is running. Add up to 1/2 cup, total, to achieve the desired pastelike consistency. If adding to pasta, toss with the cooked pasta while it is still warm.

Cauliflower "Popcorn"

FOOD GROUP(S): N/A
MEAL PLAN: 3-DAY

132 calories, 15.3 g carbohydrates, 7.3 g fat, 1.1 g saturated fat,
5.7 g protein, 7.2 g fiber, 470 mg sodium per serving

Cutting the cauliflower into such small pieces allows them to brown evenly and have a roasted flavor that is out of this world. Two heads of cauliflower may seem like a lot to start with, but you'll be amazed how quickly they cook down—and how quickly they're eaten up even before you serve them. **SERVES 4**

2 heads cauliflower

2 tablespoons extra-virgin olive oil

⅔ teaspoon salt

Preheat the oven to 425°F.

Remove the cauliflower florets from the stem and cut into grape-size pieces. In a bowl, toss the cauliflower with the olive oil and salt. Spread on a baking sheet (you may need two sheets).

Bake, tossing the cauliflower every 10 to 15 minutes. Bake for about 50 minutes, or until lightly browned.

FOOD GROUP(S): 1 STARCH
MEAL PLAN: WEEK 3

Red Chard and Quinoa Salad with Pepitas

258.7 calories, 37.7 g carbohydrates, 7.3 g fat, 1.1 g saturated fat,
10.2 g protein, 5.2 g fiber, 536.1 mg sodium per serving

Chef Phoebe Lapine shared this recipe with me recently and I begged her to let me put it in the book. I was in heaven as soon as I saw the finished product, between the color that the quinoa turned to and the soft strands of chard. The pepitas added a great crunch and I was hooked! **SERVES 4**

- 1 cup uncooked quinoa
- ½ teaspoon ground turmeric
- 1 tablespoon olive oil
- 1 bunch red chard, thick bottom stems removed and sliced thinly
- Juice of 1 lemon
- ½ teaspoon salt
- ⅛ teaspoon cayenne
- ¼ cup pepitas (pumpkin seeds)

In a small, lidded saucepan, combine the quinoa and turmeric with 2 cups of water and bring to a boil. Lower the heat to low, cover, and cook for 20 minutes, or until all the water is absorbed. Fluff with a fork and allow to rest, covered, for 10 minutes.

Meanwhile, in a large, nonstick skillet, heat the olive oil over medium-high heat. Add the chard and cook, tossing constantly, until the leaves have wilted and released a good amount of liquid, about 5 minutes.

Add the lemon juice, salt, and cayenne. Continue to simmer lightly until the chard stems are tender and the liquid has reduced by a third.

Transfer the cooked quinoa to the skillet with the chard. Toss with the chard and lemon juice until well distributed—the quinoa will turn a faint pink color.

Spoon the quinoa into a large serving bowl and garnish with the pepitas. Serve warm or at room temperature.

Stuffed Peppers

FOOD GROUP(S): 1 STARCH, 1/2 DAIRY
MEAL PLAN: WEEK 4

328 calories, 46.5 g carbohydrates, 12 g fat, 2.4 g saturated fat, 11.5 g protein, 8.7 g fiber, 697.5 mg sodium per serving

These stuffed peppers are a beautiful dish to serve. The brown rice plus the veggies add a great source of fiber, while the nuts and Parmesan cheese add an extra oomph of flavor! **SERVES 2**

1 cup cooked brown rice

½ cup chopped zucchini

½ cup chopped tomatoes

2 tablespoons pine nuts or chopped walnuts

½ teaspoon dried basil

½ teaspoon dried oregano

Salt

Freshly ground black pepper

1 cup plus 2 tablespoons marinara sauce (approved brand; see page 238)

2 bell peppers, tops removed and seeded

2 tablespoons grated Parmesan cheese

Mix the brown rice with the zucchini and tomatoes, nuts, herbs, salt and pepper to taste, and 2 tablespoons of the marinara sauce, then fill the peppers with mixture.

Place the peppers in a single layer on the bottom of a large saucepan, surround with the remaining cup of marinara sauce, cover, and simmer until warmed through and the peppers are soft, 20 to 30 minutes.

Sprinkle with grated parmesan and serve immediately.

FOOD GROUP(S): 1 STARCH
MEAL PLAN: WEEK 3
Vegetarian "Bolognese"

102.8 calories, 11 g carbohydrates, 3.9 g fat, 0.5 g saturated fat,
2.8 g protein, 2.5 g fiber, 624.8 mg sodium per serving

Who needs meat, when you have a dish like this? Sure to please any carnivore, this "meaty" sauce is great over not only pasta but also greens, such as sautéed spinach or kale, to make it Week 2 friendly.
SERVES 4

- 1 tablespoon olive oil
- 1 medium-size onion, chopped
- 1 medium-size carrot, chopped
- 8 ounces mushrooms, chopped finely
- 1 large tomato, chopped (with liquid, about 1 cup)
- ½ cup dry red wine
- 1 teaspoon dried parsley
- 2 tablespoons tomato paste
- 1 teaspoon salt
- Freshly ground black pepper
- 8 ounces whole wheat penne (see approved-brand pasta, page 237), cooked
- Freshly grated Parmesan or pecorino cheese, for garnish (optional)

In a large skillet, heat the olive oil and sauté the carrot and onion until the onion turns translucent, about 5 minutes. Add the mushrooms and cook for another 5 minutes. Stir in the chopped tomato and tomato paste, red wine, parsley, salt, and pepper to taste. Simmer until the sauce thickens, about 20 minutes.

Serve with the cooked penne (½ cup per person). Top with grated Parmesan or pecorino, if desired.

Snacks

FOOD GROUP(S): N/A
MEAL PLAN: 3-DAY

Sweetish Nuts

192.2 calories, 5.9 g carbohydrates, 54.9 g fat, 6.2 g saturated fat,
12.2 g protein, 6.1 g fiber, 4.8 mg sodium per serving

Although these nuts are sugar free, they have a natural sweetness
that comes out thanks to the cinnamon, ginger, and vanilla. Leave
a bowl of them on your counter and see how quickly they disappear! **SERVES 12**

    1½ teaspoons ground cinnamon
    1 teaspoon ground ginger
    1½ teaspoons vanilla extract
    1½ teaspoons extra-virgin olive oil
    4 ounces shelled raw walnut halves
    4 ounces shelled raw pecan halves
    4 ounces raw cashews

Preheat the oven to 325°F. Mix the cinnamon, ginger, vanilla, and olive
oil in a large bowl. Add the nuts and massage in the spices well. Place
on a baking sheet and bake for 10 to 12 minutes. Once cooled, nuts can
be stored in an airtight container.

FOOD GROUP(S): N/A
MEAL PLAN: 3-DAY

Sage Pork Jerky

75.9 calories, 0.1 g carbohydrates, 1.3 g fat, 0.4 g saturated fat,
13.5 g protein, 0 g fiber, 449.4 mg sodium per serving

It's hard to find a packaged jerky without any added sugar, so we decided to make our own. This simple recipe packs a big flavor punch
without being loaded in sugar or preservatives! **SERVES 8**

1 pound pork loin, sliced thinly

3 tablespoons soy sauce

2 tablespoons red wine

2 tablespoons finely chopped fresh sage

Preheat the oven to 200°F. Combine all the ingredients and marinate for 2 hours. Lay out the pork on a baking sheet and bake until dried, rotating the pork every 30 minutes for approximately 2 hours.

Slow-Roasted Cherry Tomatoes

FOOD GROUP(S): N/A
MEAL PLAN: WEEK 1

87.5 calories, 2 g carbohydrates, 7.2 g fat, 1 g saturated fat, 1.2 g protein, 1.2 g fiber, 295.5 mg sodium per serving

Chef Phoebe shares another fan favorite recipe of hers. These should be the real nature's candy instead of raisins. It's amazing how quickly they disappear by people passing through the kitchen. We were excited to have some left over that we used to scramble with some eggs! **SERVES 2**

1 quart mixed cherry tomatoes, halved lengthwise

6 cloves garlic, unpeeled

1 tablespoon olive oil

¼ teaspoon sea salt

¼ teaspoon freshly ground black pepper

2 teaspoons fresh oregano leaves

Preheat the oven to 225°F.

Arrange the tomatoes on a parchment-lined baking sheet, cut side up. Nestle the garlic cloves among the tomatoes. Drizzle with the olive oil—enough so each tomato gets some, season with salt and pepper, and sprinkle the oregano leaves over the top.

Roast for 2 to 3 hours, until the tomatoes are shriveled but retain some moisture, and are sweet, sour, and unbelievably delicious.

Desserts

Dark Chocolate–Covered Strawberries

FOOD GROUP(S): 1 FRUIT, 1 CHOCOLATE
MEAL PLAN: WEEK 3

172.8 calories, 20.5 g carbohydrates, 10.3 g fat, 3.2 g saturated fat,
5.4 g protein, 4.3 g fiber, 212 mg sodium per serving

Who would have thought this classic dessert would be okay to eat on a diet? Five whole strawberries as one serving make you question if you really are following the diet at all! **SERVES 4 (5 STRAWBERRIES PER SERVING)**

3½ ounces dark chocolate (65% cacao or more), chopped
1 pound strawberries (about 20) with stems, washed and dried well

Place the chocolate in a heatproof bowl. Fill a small saucepan with a few inches of water and bring to a simmer over medium heat. Turn off the heat, set the bowl of chocolate over the water (the bottom of the bowl should not touch the water), and stir until melted and smooth. (The chocolate can also be melted in the microwave at half power for 1 minute, stirred, and then heated for another 30 seconds, or until melted.)

Line a plate or sheet pan with parchment or waxed paper. Holding a strawberry by the stem, dip the fruit into the chocolate, lift, and twist to let the excess chocolate drip off into the bowl. Set the strawberry on the prepared pan and repeat. Chill the strawberries in the refrigerator for about 30 minutes, until the chocolate sets.

Very Nutty Chocolate Bark

FOOD GROUP(S): 1 CHOCOLATE
MEAL PLAN: WEEK 3

158.2 calories, 10.3 g carbohydrates, 12.9 g fat, 5.3 g saturated fat,
3.1 g protein, 3.2 g fiber, 2.6 mg sodium per serving

This chocolate bark comes out so rich and satisfying. Macadamia nuts add a wholesomeness to this sweet treat that's incredible! **SERVES 16 (1.5 SQUARES PER SERVING)**

10½ ounces dark chocolate (65% cacao or more), chopped
½ cup unsalted macadamia nuts
½ cup unsalted almonds

Place the chocolate in a heatproof bowl. Fill a small saucepan with a few inches of water and bring to a simmer over medium heat. Turn off the heat, set the bowl of chocolate over the water (the bottom of the bowl should not touch the water), and stir until melted and smooth. (The chocolate can also be melted in the microwave at half power for 1 minute, stirred, and then heated for another 30 seconds, or until melted.)

Line a 9-by-9-inch baking pan with parchment paper. Pour two-thirds of the melted chocolate over the paper and spread evenly. Sprinkle the macadamia nuts and almonds over the chocolate and then cover with the remaining chocolate. Chill the bark in the refrigerator for at least 2 hours, or until firmly set. Remove from the pan and cut the bark into sixteen squares.

Baked Apple Pie Slices

FOOD GROUP(S): 1 FRUIT
MEAL PLAN: 3-DAY

---

109 calories, 28.3 g carbohydrates, 0.3 g fat, 0 g saturated fat,
0.6 g protein, 3.2 g fiber, 1 mg sodium per serving

The aroma that happens within five minutes of these going into the oven is mouthwatering. With the delicious addition of the vanilla, cinnamon, and cloves, this is as close to a guilt-free apple pie as one can get! Try sprinkling some crushed nuts on top for an added crunch. **SERVES 4**

4 large apples, peeled and cored
1 teaspoon vanilla extract
1 teaspoon ground cinnamon
½ teaspoon ground cloves

Preheat the oven to 350°F. Slice the apples into ½-inch-thick slices. In a bowl, mix together the vanilla, cinnamon, and cloves. Add the apples and mix well. Fill a large baking pan with ¼ inch of water and lay the spiced apples in the water in a single layer. Bake for 30 minutes, or until soft. Drain the water off and serve the apples warm.

Broiled Grapefruit

FOOD GROUP(S): 1 FRUIT
MEAL PLAN: WEEK 2

28 calories, 7.2 g carbohydrates, 0.1 g fat, 0 g saturated fat, 0.5 g protein, 1.2 g fiber, 0.3 mg sodium per serving

Plain grapefruit for dessert? Absolutely! By broiling the grapefruit, its natural sugar is brought to the forefront of each bite, making this a hot and spicy treat! **SERVES 2**

1 large grapefruit
½ teaspoon ground cinnamon

Preheat the broiler on HIGH.

Slice the grapefruit in half. Using a grapefruit knife, cut around each segment of both halves but leave in place in the skin. Sprinkle the cinnamon over the grapefruit and place under the broiler. Broil for 5 to 8 minutes, or until sizzling. Serve immediately.

Grilled Stone Fruit with Cinnamon-Spiced Ricotta Cheese

FOOD GROUP(S): ¼ DAIRY, 1 FRUIT
MEAL PLAN: WEEK 3

141.5 calories, 19.1 g carbohydrates, 6.4 g fat, 2 g saturated fat,
5.1 g protein, 2.8 g fiber, 38.5 mg sodium per serving

Grilled fruit is delicious and so easy to make. Topping it with cinnamon-spiced ricotta cheese makes it even better! **SERVES 4**

4 peaches, plums, or nectarines, halved and pitted
1 tablespoon extra-virgin olive oil
½ teaspoon ground cinnamon
½ cup part-skim ricotta cheese
Fresh mint sprigs, for garnish

Preheat a grill to medium high.

Brush the fruit with the olive oil. Place on the hot grill and grill until marks appear, 2 to 3 minutes per side. Combine the cinnamon and ricotta in a small bowl. Top each half of fruit with the ricotta mixture. Garnish with a mint sprig.

Beverages

Fruity "Sangria"

FOOD GROUP(S): 1 WINE
MEAL PLAN: WEEK 3

---

224 calories, 14.4 g carbohydrates, 0 g fat, 0 g saturated fat, 0.6 g protein, 1.3 g fiber, 0.3 mg sodium per serving

---

Red wine gets a fun little twist here in our version of a sangria without any of the added sugar! Best part is that two glasses of this drink equals only one glass of regular red wine, so enjoy safely! **SERVES 4**

- 4 cups red wine
- 4 cups seltzer
- 1 orange, sliced
- 1 lime, sliced

Mix all the ingredients together in a large pitcher. Add ice to chill to desired temperature, serve, and drink responsibly.

APPENDIX A
The 31-Day Meal Plan

If an item has an asterisk (*), turn to Chapter 13 or the Recipe Index to find its recipe. If an item is double-asterisked (**), see Appendix B for approved-brand products. Our recommended serving size for red meat, pork, chicken, turkey, fish and seafood is 6 ounces; for these proteins and eggs, vegetarians and vegans may substitute 6 ounces of tofu, or ½ cup of cooked legumes, such as lentils or beans. See page 95 for recommended serving sizes of dairy ingredients.

TABLE A.1 The 31-Day Meal Plan, Days 1–3

3-Day Sugar Fix	Day 1	Day 2	Day 3
Breakfast	3 scrambled eggs w/pinch of dried rosemary	Sautéed spinach scrambled w/3 eggs	3-egg omelet w/shrimp, sautéed spinach & tarragon
Snack	1 ounce mixed nuts	1 ounce mixed nuts	1 ounce mixed nuts
Lunch	Poached chicken on top of mixed baby greens and ½ sliced avocado with herbs, olive oil, and red wine vinegar	Tuna Niçoise (no potatoes): canned tuna, mixed greens, one hard-boiled egg, and steamed green beans, Sugar Detox Vinaigrette*	Grilled turkey burger in lettuce wrap w/sliced avocado
Snack	Sliced bell peppers, 2 tablespoons hummus	Sliced bell peppers, 2 tablespoons hummus	Sliced bell peppers, 2 tablespoons hummus
Dinner	½ cup of edamame, salmon w/stir-fried broccoli and mushrooms	Rosemary pork, sautéed Brussels sprouts, chopped romaine lettuce with avocado and lemon	Steamed chicken with ginger, soy sauce, and sesame oil; sautéed cauliflower

TABLE A.2 The 31-Day Meal Plan, Days 4–10

WEEK 1	Day 4	Day 5	Day 6	Day 7	Day 8	Day 9	Day 10
Breakfast	2 Spinach-Egg Muffins*	Greek yogurt** with 2 tablespoons slivered almonds and dash of vanilla extract; crackers**	Cottage Cheese with ½ sliced avocado	Goat cheese and spinach 3-egg omelet	2 eggs scrambled with spinach and salsa**, 2 high-fiber crackers**	Greek yogurt** with 2 tablespoons flaxseed and 1 teaspoon vanilla extract	3 eggs poached over sautéed greens
Snack	1 medium apple, 1 tablespoon almond butter	1 ounce pumpkin seeds	Crackers**, 1 tablespoon peanut butter**	Chia Seed Pudding*	Cauliflower Popcorn*	1 medium apple, sliced, 1 ounce cottage cheese, 2 high-fiber crackers**	Crackers**, 1 ounce sunflower seeds
Lunch	Mixed greens, chickpeas, feta, bell pepper, cucumbers, olive oil & balsamic vinegar; crackers**	Turkey lettuce wraps w/ Dijon mustard	Grilled chicken on top of mixed greens salad with string beans, 1 medium apple	Baked chicken with spices, Asparagus and Mushroom Salad*	6 pieces sashimi, miso soup, seaweed salad	Tuna Niçoise (see Day 2 of 3-Day plan) with olive oil & balsamic vinegar; crackers**	Chicken skewers, with hummus. lettuce cups, and carrot sticks
Snack	1 cup edamame, in the pod	1 ounce Sweetish Nuts*	Sliced cucumbers; hummus	1 ounce cashews sprinkled with cinnamon and cayenne, 1 medium apple	1 apple, 1 piece string cheese	Sliced peppers with 2 tablespoons hummus	Sage Pork Jerky*, 1 medium apple, sliced
Dinner	Spaghetti squash sautéed with garlic, olive oil, kale, peppers, and ¼ cup marinara**	Poached Chicken Breast and Zucchini Pasta*, 1 baked medium apple	Mustard Crusted Salmon*, mixed greens salad	Baked Shrimp with Spinach and Tomato*	Baked tofu topped with sesame seeds and sesame oil or soy sauce, with steamed asparagus	Poached Halibut with Ginger-Lime Sauce*	Grilled salmon with sautéed broccoli and onions

TABLE A.3 The 31-Day Meal Plan, Days 11–17

WEEK 2	Day 11	Day 12	Day 13	Day 14	Day 15	Day 16	Day 17
Breakfast	Greek yogurt** with ½ cup blueberries, plus cinnamon, flaxseeds, and walnuts	2 eggs, scrambled w/spinach;	Smoothie: 1 cup Lifeway Low-Fat plain kefir, ½ cup frozen raspberries, ¼ teaspoon vanilla extract, 1 teaspoon chia seeds	Frittata*	Greek yogurt** w/½ cup sliced strawberries and 1 tablespoon sliced almonds	1 medium apple, 1.5 tablespoons peanut butter**, and cinnamon	2-egg omelet w/mushrooms and 1 tablespoon shredded Parmesan, 2 high-fiber crackers**
Snack	Crackers**, w/avocado and lemon	1 medium apple, sliced, over cottage cheese	1 medium apple, 1 ounce cashews	1 medium apple, 1 tablespoon almond butter	12 cherry tomatoes drizzled with balsamic vinegar	Plain yogurt** w/vanilla extract, cinnamon, and 1 ounce almonds	Sliced peppers; Curried Yogurt Dip: Greek yogurt** w/curry powder and salt
Lunch	2 cups arugula, 1 can tuna in water, ½ bell pepper, 6 olives, lemon vinaigrette	Kidney beans tossed w/cumin, garlic and chile powder, diced avocado and tomato, lime juice, and oil served over red leaf lettuce and topped w/cilantro; crackers**	½ cup chickpeas, 1 tablespoon crumbled feta, ½ tomato diced, ¼ cup black olives, baby spinach, and red wine vinaigrette	2 Wasa crackers**, ¼ avocado smashed, canned tuna** w/extra-virgin olive oil and lemon juice, and capers; large green salad w/cucumber and tomato	1 cup Garlic Soup*, 2 Wasa crackers** w/1 ounce goat cheese and sliced cucumber; 1 medium apple	1 cup gazpacho, grilled chicken	Kale salad w/¼ cup hummus, carrots, bell pepper, 1 tablespoon chopped walnuts, and red wine vinaigrette

Snack	String cheese and 1 medium apple	Yogurt** topped w/ blueberries and 1 ounce roasted pumpkin seeds	Sliced bell pepper and 1 ounce sharp Cheddar cheese	½ cup blueberries, 1 ounce almonds	Celery sticks w/1 tablespoon peanut butter**, 1 ounce cashews	Cantaloupe, sliced, with cottage cheese, crackers**	½ cup raspberries, 1 ounce pistachios
Dinner	Sautéed chicken w/ peppers, onions and marinara sauce; small mixed green salad	1 cup steamed string beans, 2 grilled shrimp and zucchini kebabs	Pan-seared pork chop; 2 cups sautéed kale w/ garlic	Chicken "Fajitas" in Lettuce Wraps*	Sushi Night: 6 pieces sashimi; 1 cup miso soup, small seaweed salad	Grilled salmon; 1 cup steamed asparagus; small arugula salad	Stuffed Bell Pepper*, 6 ounces filet mignon

TABLE A.4 The 31-Day Meal Plan, Days 18–24

WEEK 3	Day 18	Day 19	Day 20	Day 21	Day 22	Day 23	Day 24
Breakfast	Greek yogurt** topped with sliced apple and ground flaxseeds	½ cup cooked oatmeal with blueberries and hemp seeds	Crackers** topped with 1 tablespoon peanut butter** and sliced apple; café au lait (brewed coffee plus ½ cup warm low-fat milk)	2-egg omelet with asparagus, 1 slice Canadian bacon	Greek yogurt** with 1 peach, sliced, 2 high-fiber crackers**	Scrambled eggs w/lox (2 eggs, 1 ounce lox) and sliced tomato	2 eggs, sunny-side up, 2 cups sautéed kale with olive oil, oregano, and hot pepper flakes (optional)
Snack	Sliced strawberries over cottage cheese	Sliced cucumber, 1 ounce goat cheese, 2 high-fiber crackers**	Chia Seed Pudding* topped w/ berries	Carrots with 2 tablespoons Curried Yogurt Dip: Greek yogurt** w/curry powder and salt	1 ounce Sweetish Nuts*	1 ounce almonds	Sage Pork Jerky*, 1 medium apple, sliced
Lunch	Black bean chili, bell pepper strips, crackers**	Turkey burger wrapped in lettuce and topped with salsa and avocado, mixed green salad	Buckwheat noodles stir-fried with tofu, bean sprouts, cauliflower, sesame oil, soy sauce, and hot pepper flakes	½ cup whole wheat pasta with tomato sauce**; mix in chopped onion, pepper, mushrooms, 2 tablespoons flaxseed; baked chicken breast, 1 ounce dark chocolate	Salad with ½ cup chickpeas, shredded carrots, cucumbers, and mustard dressing	Poached Halibut with Ginger Lime Sauce*, ½ cup cooked quinoa, small salad	Curried Chicken Salad: Chicken breast, chopped, mixed w/ ½ cup sliced grapes, ¼ cup Greek yogurt**, and 1 teaspoon curry powder, in lettuce wraps

Snack	Sliced cucumber and carrot with hummus	1 medium apple, Greek yogurt** w/ cinnamon	1 hard-boiled egg, sliced, w/ crackers** and hummus	Smoked salmon with 1 ounce goat cheese, 2 high-fiber crackers**	1 orange, 1 wedge Laughing Cow cheese	2 small clementines, 1 ounce cashews, 1 ounce dark chocolate	1 peach, sliced, and cottage cheese
Dinner	Asparagus and Mushroom Salad*, baked scallops, 1/2 cup cooked quinoa; 1 ounce dark chocolate	Steak, Haricots Verts with Mint*, Dark Chocolate–Covered Strawberries*	Baked shrimp with lemon and pepper, mixed green salad, 1 ounce dark chocolate	Braised Short Ribs* string bean salad	Veggie burger with 1/4 avocado, tomato slices, wrapped in lettuce, 1 ounce dark chocolate	Curried lentil soup, cucumber and tomato salad, 2 high-fiber crackers**	Sautéed chicken and mushrooms over 1/2 cup cooked brown rice, arugula salad, Very Nutty Chocolate Bark*

TABLE A.5 The 31-Day Meal Plan, Days 25–31

WEEK 4	Day 25	Day 26	Day 27	Day 28	Day 29	Day 30	Day 31
Breakfast	Cottage Cheese Pancakes*, 1 ounce chopped almonds, 1 peach, sliced	2 eggs, sunny-side up, 2 cups spinach sautéed with coconut oil	¾ cup Uncle Sam cereal**, w/½ cup almond milk**, ½ cup blueberries	½ cup plain cooked oatmeal, ½ cup mixed berries, 2 tablespoons flaxseeds	1 cup Kashi Whole Grain Puffs**, ½ cup almond milk**, 1 medium apple	2 Spinach-Egg Muffins*, 2 slices turkey bacon	Greek yogurt** w/2 tablespoons flaxseeds and ½ cup halved grapes
Snack	1 cup yogurt** w/chopped apple	Kale chips**	1 tablespoon almond butter** and 1 medium apple, sliced	Crackers** with 1 tbsp peanut butter	2 high-fiber crackers** spread with ¼ avocado	1 small baked sweet potato (about ½ cup), sprinkled w/ cinnamon	2 high-fiber crackers** with tuna and a little mayo
Lunch	½ avocado salad stuffed with tuna and Sugar Detox Vinaigrette*, crackers**	Turkey Meatballs in Marinara Sauce*, ½ cup whole wheat pasta**	Turkey on a whole-grain tortilla** topped with mustard, tomato, and lettuce	Greek salad with grilled shrimp, ½ cup grapes	Mustard Crusted Salmon*, sautéed snap peas and onions	Black Bean Salad*, served with sautéed greens and ½ cup yogurt**	Cajun Dirty Brown Rice*
Snack	Slow-Roasted Cherry Tomatoes*	½ grapefruit, 1 ounce pistachios	1 cup cantaloupe, 1 Laughing Cow wedge	1 hard-boiled egg, halved & topped with 1 tbsp hummus	½ cup strawberries w/ricotta cheese and cinnamon	2 high-fiber crackers, *1 wedge Laughing Cow cheese, cherry tomatoes	2 clementines, 1 ounce roasted pumpkin seeds

Dinner						
Poached white fish with ratatouille; Very Nutty Chocolate Bark*	Guacamole with sliced jicama, open-faced lean beef burger on ½ English muffin**; 1 baked medium apple w/cinnamon	Baked Shrimp with Spinach and Tomato* ½ cup cooked brown rice; Skip dessert today	Chicken Fajitas*, 1 tortilla**; Grilled Stone Fruit w/Ricotta Cheese*	Poached scallops on bed of sautéed kale; 1 ounce dark chocolate	Poached Chicken Breasts* with Zucchini Pasta*; Baked Apple Pie Slices*	Turkey (or soy) sausage, ½ cup quinoa mixed with chopped kale, olive oil, seasoning; Fruity Sangria*; Skip dessert today

APPENDIX B
Approved-Brand Foods

These brand-name packaged products are fine to add to your diet during and after the stated period that follows; for example, an item designated "Week 3" may be consumed during Weeks 3 and 4, and thereafter during Maintenance. See Chapter 1 for more about daily allowances and serving sizes.

Brooke's Favorite Finds

Barney Butter Almond Butter	3-Day
Doctor in the Kitchen Rosemary Flackers Flax Seed Crackers	3-Day
Explore Asian Organic Mung Bean Pasta	Week 1
LaCroix Sparkling Water (all flavors)	3-Day
Madecasse Madagascar Chocolat (Exotic Pepper, 70% Cacao, 75% Cacao, or 80% Cacao)	Week 3
Mary's Gone Crackers (Original, Black Pepper, Caraway, Herb, or Onion)	Week 3
Nature's Path Qi'a cereal	3-Day
Quinn Popcorn (Parmesan & Rosemary or Lemon & Sea Salt)	Week 1
Sea Tangle Kelp Noodles	3-Day
Sheffa Savory Bars Rosemary Savory Bar	Week 4
Sweetriot 65% dark chocolate covered cacao nibs	Week 3
Teas' Tea, Unsweetened (all flavors)	3-Day
Wild Squirrel Curious Cocoa-Nut Chocolate Coconut Peanut Butter	3-Day

Breads/Crackers/Wraps

The Baker Bread, Organic (Whole Grain, Flax Seed, or Sunflower Seed)	Week 3
Back to Nature Harvest Whole Wheat Crackers	Week 3
Brad's Raw Flax Crackers (Sun Dried Tomato)	Week 1
Ezekiel Bread	Week 3
Finn Crisp Hi-Fibre	Week 1
GG Crackers	Week 1
Kashi Heart to Heart Whole Grain Crackers (Original or Roasted Garlic)	Week 3
La Tortilla Factory SoftWraps (all varieties)	Week 3
Lydia's Organics Sunflower Seed Bread	Week 3
Mestemacher Bread (Fitness, Muesli, Natural Rye & Spelt, or Whole Rye)	Week 3
Old London Melba Toast, Whole Grain	Week 3
Orgran Crispbread with Quinoa	Week 3
Ryvita Crispbread (Light Rye or Sunflower Seeds and Oats)	Week 3
Silver Hills Sprouted Bakery Steady Eddie Bread	Week 3
Toufayan Pitettes and Mini Pitettes, Whole Wheat	Week 3
Toufayan Lavash, Multigrain	Week 3
Triscuits Whole Grain Crackers	Week 1
Two Moms in the Raw Sea Crackers (Pesto or Tomato Basil)	Week 3
Vermont Bread Company Bread (Sodium Free Whole Wheat Bread, Soft 10 Grain, or Soft Whole Wheat	Week 3
Wasa Crispbread (Hearty Rye or Light Rye)	Week 3
Whole Foods Organic English Muffins (Multigrain or Wheat)	Week 3

Cereal

365 Organic Multi Grain and Flax Instant Oatmeal	Week 3
Arrowhead Mills Organic Oat Bran Flakes	Week 3
Arrowhead Mills Organic Spelt Flakes	Week 3
Arrowhead Mills Puffed Wheat	Week 3
Arrowhead Mills Shredded Wheat	Week 3
Barbara's Shredded Wheat	Week 3
Cascadian Farm Organic Purely O's	Week 3
Ezekiel Sprouted Whole Grain Cereal (Original, Almond, or Golden Flax)	Week 3
General Mills Cheerios	Week 3

General Mills Fiber One, Original	Week 3
General Mills Wheaties	Week 3
Kashi 7 Whole Grain Nuggets or Puffs	Week 3
Kellogg's Corn Flakes	Week 3
Kellogg's Product 19	Week 3
Kellogg's Special K (Original or Protein Plus)	Week 3
Nature's Path Organic Flax Plus, Multibran	Week 3
Nature's Path Organic Heritage (Original, Bites, or O's)	Week 3
Nature's Path Organic Oatbran (Millet Rice or Multigrain)	Week 3
Nature's Path Organic Synergy	Week 3
Nutritious Living Hi-Lo (Maple Pecan or Vanilla Almond)	Week 3
Old Wessex Oatmeal	Week 3
Post Grape-Nuts (Original or Flakes)	Week 3
Post (or any brand) Shredded Wheat (Original, Original Spoon Size, or Wheat 'n Bran)	Week 3
Umpqua Oats Not Guilty	Week 3
Uncle Sam (Original or with Real Mixed Berries)	Week 3
Weetabix Organic Crispy Flakes	Week 3

Chocolate

Green & Black's	Week 3
NibMor	Week 3
Sweet Riot Flavor 70	Week 3

Desserts

So Delicious Organic No-Sugar-Added Coconut Milk Ice Cream (Chocolate, Vanilla Bean, Mint Chip, or Toasted Almond Chip)

Fish

Any brand canned or jarred tuna	3-Day
Wild Planet Wild Alaskan Salmon (Pink or Sockeye)	3-Day
Wild Planet Wild Albacore Tuna Fillets (Original or in Extra-Virgin Olive Oil)	3-Day
Wild Planet Wild California Sardines (in Spring Water, in Extra-Virgin Olive Oil, or with Lemon)	3-Day
Wild Planet Wild Pink Shrimp	3-Day
Wild Planet Wild Skipjack Light Tuna	3-Day

Frozen Meals

Amy's Bowls (Brown Rice, Black-Eyed Peas, or Veggies)	Week 4
Amy's Indian Spinach Tofu Burrito	Week 4
Birds Eye Steamfresh frozen vegetables	3-Day
Deep Indian Gourmet Dal Masala Curry	3-Day
Ethnic Gourmet Chicken Tandoori with Spinach	3-Day
Ethnic Gourmet Palak Paneer	Week 1
Kashi Three Cheese Penne	Week 4
Kashi Pesto Pasta Primavera	Week 4
Tandoor Chef Channa Masala	3-Day
Whole Foods 365 Organic Roasted Vegetable Pizza (Whole Wheat)	Week 4

Meat

Applegate Organics Chicken and Turkey Sausage (Fire Roasted Red Pepper or Sweet Italian)	3-Day
Applegate Organics Chicken and Turkey Sausage in Spinach and Feta	Week 1
Applegate Organics Herb Turkey Breast	3-Day
Applegate Organics Roast Beef	3-Day
Applegate Organics Uncured Hot Dogs (Beef, Chicken, or Turkey)	3-Day
Applegate Organics Smoked Turkey Breast	3-Day
Great Range Ground Bison	3-Day
Jennie-O All Natural Turkey Burgers	3-Day
Wellshire Smoked Andouille Sausage	3-Day

Meat Substitutes

Boca All-American Classic Meatless Burger	Week 3
De Canto's Best Burger (Original, Garlic, or Quinoa)	Week 3
Gardenburger The Original Veggie Burger	Week 3
Sunshine Burgers, Garden Herb	Week 3

Milk/Milk Alternatives

Almond Breeze Almond Milk, Unsweetened (Original or Chocolate)	Week 1
Organic Valley Organic Omega-3 Milk	Week 1

Organic Eden Soy Milk, Unsweetened	Week 1
Pacific Organic Almond Milk, Unsweetened (Original or Vanilla)	Week 1
So Delicious Almond Plus, Original	Week 1
So Delicious Coconut Milk, Original Sugar-free	Week 1
Tempt Hemp Milk, Original Unsweetened	Week 1
West Soy Organic Soy Milk, Unsweetened	Week 1

Nut Butters/Spreads

Any unsweetened, unsalted nut butters	3-Day
Maple Grove Farms Peanut Butter (Crunchy or Creamy)	3-Day
Naturally More Peanut Butter (Crunchy or Creamy)	3-Day
Peanut Butter Co. Old Fashioned Smooth Peanut Butter	3-Day
Smuckers Natural Peanut Butter (Crunchy or Creamy)	3-Day
Sunbutter, Organic Unsweetened	3-Day

Pastas/Grains/Noodles

Annie Chun's Rice Express Sprouted Brown Sticky Rice	Week 4
Barilla Plus Pastas	Week 3
Bionaturae 100% Whole Wheat Pastas	Week 3
Casablanca Gardens Whole Wheat Couscous	Week 3
DeCecco 100% Whole Wheat Pastas (Fusilli, Linguine, Penne Rigate, Spaghetti)	Week 3
Eden Organic Pasta Kamut Spirals	Week 3
Einkorn Spaghetti	Week 3
Explore Asian Organic Blackbean Spaghetti	3-Day
Explore Asian Organic Soybean Spaghetti	Week 3
Hodgson Mill Whole Wheat Macaroni & Cheese Dinner	Week 3
Lundberg Country Wild Whole Grain Brown Rice	Week 4
Minute Instant Whole Grain Brown Rice	Week 3
Near East Whole Grain Chicken and Herb Rice	Week 4
Rice Select Pearl Couscous, Whole Wheat	Week 3
Ronzoni Healthy Harvest 100% Whole Grain Pastas	Week 3
Uncle Ben's Ready Rice Whole Grain Brown Rice	Week 4

Salad Dressings

Annie's Naturals Organic (Oil and Vinegar, Goddess, Shiitake & Sesame, or Tuscany Italian)	Week 1

Brianna's Home Style Real French Vinaigrette	Week 1
Newman's Own (Olive Oil & Vinegar or Caesar)	Week 1

Salsas and Other Dips

Amy's Salsa (Mild or Medium)	Week 1
D.L. Jardines Salsa (Cilantro Green Olive or Texacante)	Week 1
Green Mountain Gringo Salsa (Mild or Roasted Chile Pepper)	Week 1
Muir Glen Organic Salsa (Garden Cilantro or Mild)	Week 1
Wholly Guacamole (Classic, Avocado Verde, Guacamole & Spicy Pico, Homestyle, Organic, or Spicy)	Week 1
Wholly Salsa (Mild, Medium, or Hot)	Week 1

Sauces

Cholula Hot Sauce	3-Day
Amy's Family Marinara Sauce	Week 1
Classico Sauce (Spicy Red Pepper or Tomato and Basil)	Week 1
Louisiana The Original Hot Sauce	3-Day
Miso Master Organic Miso (Original or Mellow White)	3-Day
Miso Master Organic Miso (Brown Rice, Country Barley, or Organic Red)	Week 3
Muir Glen Organic Tomato Sauce	Week 1
Prego Marinara Sauce	Week 1
Rao's Homemade Sauce (Arrabbiata, Garden Vegetable, Marinara, Puttanesca, Roasted Eggplant Sauce, Sensitive Formula Marinara, or Tomato Basil)	Week 1
Tabasco Sauce	3-Day

Snacks

365 Organic Applesauce, Unsweetened	Week 1
479° Popcorn (Black Truffle + White Cheddar)	Week 1
Bare Fruit 100% Organic Bake-Dried Cinnamon Apple Chips	Week 1
Brad's Raw Leafy Kale (Naked)	3-Day
cruncha ma-me Edamame Snacks	1 Day
Danielle Spicy Carrot Chips	Week 2
Good Health Half Naked Popcorn	Week 1

Nature's All Foods Freeze Dried Strawberries	Week 2
Nutty Bean Co. ChickPz, Sea Salt	3-Day
Seapoint Farms Dry Roasted Edamame	3-Day
SeaSnax Lightly Roasted and Seasoned Seaweed Snack	3-Day
Skinny Pop Popcorn	Week 1
Sunbiotics Almonds (Original, Cheesy or Truffle)	3-Day

Soups

Amy's Curried Red Lentil	Week 1
Amy's Low Fat, Split Pea	Week 2
Amy's Low Fat Vegetable Barley	Week 3
Tabatchnick Split Pea Soup (Low Sodium, not the organic one)	Week 2

Veggies

Birds Eye Steamfresh frozen vegetables	3-Day
Mann's California Stir Fry	3-Day
Mann's Rainbow Salad	3-Day

Yogurt

Brown Cow Smooth and Creamy Greek Yogurt, Plain	Week 1
Chobani Nonfat, Plain	Week 1
Fage Total 2%, Plain	Week 1
The Greek Gods Nonfat Greek Yogurt, Plain	Week 1
Stonyfield Organic Oikos Greek Yogurt, Plain	Week 1
Siggi's Skyr Yogurt, Plain	Week 1
Voskos Organic Nonfat Greek Style Yogurt, Plain	Week 1
Yoplait Greek 2% Fat 2x Protein Yogurt, Plain	Week 1
Lifeway Low-Fat Plain Kefir	Week 1

Miscellaneous

Any brand unsweetened cocoa powder	3-Day
Laughing Cow cheeses	Week 1
Oloves (Tasty Mediterranean, Hot Chilli Mama, or Lemony Lover)	Week 1

APPENDIX C
Suggested Skin Care Products

TABLE C.1 Suggested Products

	Product	Description	Skin Type
Cleansers	CeraVe Hydrating Cleanser	Ceramide, hyaluronic acid	Normal to dry
	CeraVe Foaming Facial Cleanser	Ceramide, hyaluronic acid, niacinamide	Normal to oily
	Cetaphil Gentle Skin Cleanser for all skin types	Gentle soap-free cleanser Use with or without water	All skin types including sensitive
	Cetaphil DermaControl Foam Wash	Foaming cleanser with zinc	Oily acne-prone
	Effaclar Purifying Foaming Gel	Soap-free cleansing gel with zinc PCA	Oily-acne prone
	Neutrogena Naturals Purifying Facial Cleanser	Gentle cleanser with willowbark	Normal to acne prone
	Olay Foaming Face Wash— Sensitive Skin	Soap-free, oil-free, glycerin cleanser	All skin types including sensitive
	La Roche Posay Toleriane Dermo Cleanser	Gentle glycerin based cleanser	Sensitive
	Glycolix Elite Ultra Gentle Cleanser	Soap-free cleanser with vitamin A, C, E, green tea and co-enzyme Q10.	All skin types including sensitive
	Neutrogena Ultra Gentle Daily Cleanser	Mild cleanser	All skin types including sensitive
	Aveeno Positively Radiant brightening cleanser	Soy Extract	All skin types
	Keihls ultra facial cleanser for all skin types	Squalane, apricot kernel oil, vitamin E, avocado oil	All skin types
	GlyDerm Gentle Face Cleanser	Glycolic acid	All skin types

	Product	Description	Skin Type
	SkinCeuticals Purifying Cleanser	Glycolic acid gel cleanser	All skin types
	SkinCeuticals Simply Clean	Mixed alpha hydroxy acids, aloe and chamomile extract	Normal to combination
	SkinCeuticals LHA Cleansing Gel	Lipohydroxy acid, glycolic acid and salicylic acid	Normal to oily (not sensitive)
	MD formulations facial cleanser	Glycolic acid	All skin types
	NeoStrata Facial Cleanser	Gluconolactone	All skin types
	NeoStrata Skin Active Exfoliating Wash	Gluconolactone and maltobionic acid	All skin types
	Glytone acne treatment facial cleanser	Salicylic acid and glycolic acid	Oily/acne prone
	Aveeno Clear Complexion Foaming Cleanser	Salicylic acid and soy extracts	Combination to oily
	Neutrogena Oil-Free Acne Wash Pink Grapefruit Facial Cleanser	Salicylic Acid, vitamin C grapefruit extract	Oily/ acne prone
	Obagi CLENZiderm M.D. Daily Care Foaming Cleanser	Salicylic acid, menthol	Oily/ acne prone
Daily protection serums/ creams with antioxidants	Vivitè Daily Antioxidant Facial Serum	Extracts including green tea, pomegranate, chamomile, olive leaf, licorice root and glycolic acid	All skin types
	Olay Regenerist Regenerating serum	Niacinamide, green tea and pomegranate extract, carnosine, vitamin E, Matrixyl	All skin types
	La Roche-Posay Derm AOX Intensive Anti-Wrinkle Radiance Serum	Carnosine, pycnogenol, vitamin C&E	All skin types
	SkinCeuticals Phloretin CF serum	Phloretin, vitamin C, ferulic acid	All skin types
	SkinCeuticals A.G.E. Interrupter cream	Blueberry extract, Proxylane™, phytosphingosine.	Normal/dry
	Dr Dennis Gross Hydra-Pure Firming Serum	Retinol, vitamins C&E, co-enzyme Q10, peptides, extracts of green tea, tomato, grape seed and soy.	All skin types

	Product	Description	Skin Type
	NeoStrata Skin Active Antioxidant Defense Serum	Bionic and polyhydroxy acids, retinol, vitamin C and E, citric acid, extracts of green tea, chardonnay grape seed, tomato and lilac.	All skin types
	B Kamins Laboratories C-Resveratrol Serum Kx	Resveratrol, vitamin C and E, Carnosine, acai oil, coenzyme Q10, peptides	All skin types
	Korres Quercetin and Oak Antiaging and Antiwrinkle Face Serum	Quercus Robur bark extract, vitamins C and E, peptides, and Quercetin	All skin types
	OleHenriksen truth serum collagen booster	Vitamin C and E, extracts of green tea, orange fruit, rose-hips, and grapefruit seed	All skin types
	Algenist Concentrated Reconstructing Serum	Extracts of algae, swiss apple stem cell, green tea, orange, lemon. Algae exopolysaccharides, niacinamide and peptides	All skin types
	fresh Black Tea Age-Delay Serum	Extracts of black tea, blackberry leaf, rosemary leaf	All skin types
	Topix Replenix Serum CF	Green tea, caffeine, hyaluronic acid	All skin types
	Topix Replenix Power of 3 Cream or Serum	Green Tea, resveratrol, caffeine, hyaluronic acid	All skin types
	SkinMedica Rejuvenative Moisturizer	Essential fatty acids, botanical extracts, algae extract, vitamin A, C and E	All skin types
Daily moisturizers with SPF	La Roche-Posay Anthelios 60 Ultra Light Sunscreen Fluid with Cell-OX Shield XL	Avobenzone, homosalate, octisalate, octocrylene oxybenzone, botanical antioxidants	Normal to combination
	CeraVe Facial Moisturizing Lotion AM SPF 30	Homosalate, octinate, octocrylene, zinc oxide	All skin types including dry
	Cetaphil Daily Facial Moisturizer UVA/ UVB with sunscreen SPF 50	Oxtinoxate, Octisalate, Octocrylene, oxybenzone, titanium dioxide	Normal/dry
	Cetaphil DermaControl Oil Control Moisturizer SPF 30	Avobenzone, octocrylene, octisalate	Oily/acne prone

	Product	Description	Skin Type
	Clinique Super City Block Oil-Free Daily Face Protector SPF 40	Titanium dioxide, methoxycinnamate, vitamin C, E licorice extract	All skin types including oily
	Aveeno Positively Radiant Daily Moisturizer Broad Spectrum SPF 30	Avobenzone, octocrylene, oxybenzone, soy	All skin types including oily
	Eucerin Daily Protection SPF 30 Moisturizing Face Lotion	Ensulizole, octinoxate, octisalate, zinc and titanium dioxide, fragrance-free	All skin types
	Neutrogena Healthy Defense Daily Moisturizer with sunscreen Broad Spectrum SPF 50	Avobenzone, homosalate,octisalate octocrylene,oxybenzone	All skin types
	Vivitè Daily Facial Moisturizer with Sunscreen SPF 30	Octinoxate, oxybenzone, octisalate, glycolic acid, pomegranate, vitamin E and C, green tea, licorice root and olive leaf extracts, superoxide dismutase	All skin types
	Neutrogena Healthy Defense Daily Moisturizer with Sunscreen SPF 50 for Sensitive Skin	Titanium and Zinc oxide	All skin types including sensitive
	Elta MD UV Physical Broad Spectrum SPF 41	Zinc oxide, titanium dioxide (tinted)	All skin types
	SkinCeuticals Physical fusion UV defense SPF50	Zinc Oxide	All skin types
Night repair	Roc Retinol Correxion Sensitive Night Cream	Retinol-slow release	Normal to Sensitive
	Neutrogena Healthy Skin Anti-Wrinkle Cream Night	Retinol, pro-vitamin B5 and vitamin E	Normal /combination
	La Roche Posay Redermic [R] Intensive Anti-Aging Corrective Treatment	Retinol	All skin types
	SkinCeuticals Retinol 0.5 Refining Night Cream or SkinCeuticals Retinol 1.0 Refining Night Cream	Retinol Retinol	All skin types
	SkinMedica Age Defense Tri-retinol Complex or Tri-retinol Complex ES	Retinol blend, vitamin C blend vitamin and E.	All skin types ES not for sensitive

Product	Description	Skin Type
Olay Regenerist Wrinkle Revolution Complex	Matrixyl, green tea extract, niacinamide, vitamin C, vitamin B5 and E	Normal/combination
Olay Professional ProX Deep Wrinkle Treatment	Niacinamide, retinyl proprionate, vitamin E, Matrixyl and other peptides	Normal/combination
Olay Regenerist Micro-Sculpting Cream	Niacinamide, Matrixyl, dill and green tea extract	Normal to sensitive
NIA 24 Skin-Strengthening Complex Repair Cream	Pro-niacin, retinyl palmitate, green tea and rosemary extract, peptide complex	All skin types
NeoStrata Skin Active Firming Collagen Booster	Matrixyl 3000 peptide, Neoglucosamine, gardenia cell culture extract	All skin types
La Roche Posay Active C	Vitamin C, with glycerin	All skin types
Jan Marini C-ESTA Face Cream	Vitamin C blend, vitamin E, rosemary extract	All skin types
NeoStrata Ultra Moisturizing Face Cream	Gluconolactone, vitamin E	All skin types
NeoStrata Bionic Face Cream	Gluconolactone, Lactobionic acid	All skin types
NeoStrata Skin Active Cellular Restoration	Maltobioinic acid, gluconolactone, glycolic acid, peptides, extracts including grape seed, swiss apple stem cell extract, pomegranate, blueberry and vitamin E	All skin types
SkinCeuticals Renew Overnight Dry	Hydroxy blend, comfrey, aloe and chamomile extract, evening primrose oil	Normal to dry
SkinMedica AHA/BHA Cream	A blend of naturally derived alpha and beta hydroxy acids	All skin types
Vivitè Night Renewal Facial Cream	Glycolic acid, peptides, algae extract, antioxidants including vitamin C, E and superoxide dismutase, olive leaf extract	Normal/dry

METRIC CONVERSIONS

The recipes in this book have not been tested with metric measurements, so some variations might occur. Remember that the weight of dry ingredients varies according to the volume or density factor: 1 cup of flour weighs far less than 1 cup of sugar, and 1 tablespoon doesn't necessarily hold 3 teaspoons.

GENERAL FORMULA FOR METRIC CONVERSION

Ounces to grams	multiply ounces by 28.35
Grams to ounces	multiply ounces by 0.035
Pounds to grams	multiply pounds by 453.5
Pounds to kilograms	multiply pounds by 0.45
Cups to liters	multiply cups by 0.24
Fahrenheit to Celsius	subtract 32 from Fahrenheit temperature, multiply by 5, divide by 9
Celsius to Fahrenheit	multiply Celsius temperature by 9, divide by 5, add 32

VOLUME (LIQUID) MEASUREMENTS

1 teaspoon	= ⅙ fluid ounce	= 5 milliliters
1 tablespoon	= ½ fluid ounce	= 15 milliliters
2 tablespoons	= 1 fluid ounce	= 30 milliliters
¼ cup	= 2 fluid ounces	= 60 milliliters
⅓ cup	= 2⅔ fluid ounces	= 79 milliliters
½ cup	= 4 fluid ounces	= 118 milliliters
1 cup or ½ pint	= 8 fluid ounces	= 250 milliliters
2 cups or 1 pint	= 16 fluid ounces	= 500 milliliters
4 cups or 1 quart	= 32 fluid ounces	= 1,000 milliliters
1 gallon	= 4 liters	

WEIGHT (MASS) MEASUREMENTS

1 ounce	= 30 grams	
2 ounces	= 55 grams	
3 ounces	= 85 grams	
4 ounces	= ¼ pound	= 125 grams
8 ounces	= ½ pound	= 240 grams
12 ounces	= ¾ pound	= 375 grams
16 ounces	= 1 pound	= 454 grams

OVEN TEMPERATURE EQUIVALENTS, FAHRENHEIT (F) AND CELSIUS (C)

100°F	= 38°C
200°F	= 95°C
250°F	= 120°C
300°F	= 150°C
350°F	= 180°C
400°F	= 205°C
450°F	= 230° C

VOLUME (DRY) MEASUREMENTS

¼ teaspoon	= 1 milliliter
½ teaspoon	= 2 milliliters
¾ teaspoon	= 4 milliliters
1 teaspoon	= 5 milliliters
1 tablespoon	= 15 milliliters
¼ cup	= 59 milliliters
⅓ cup	= 79 milliliters
½ cup	= 118 milliliters
⅔ cup	= 158 milliliters
¾ cup	= 177 milliliters
1 cup	= 225 milliliters
4 cups or 1 quart	= 1 liter
½ gallon	= 2 liters
1 gallon	= 4 liters

LINEAR MEASUREMENTS

½ in	= 1½ cm
1 inch	= 2½ cm
6 inches	= 15 cm
8 inches	= 20 cm
10 inches	= 25 cm
12 inches	= 30 cm
20 inches	= 50 cm

ACKNOWLEDGMENTS

This book would have never been written if it hadn't been for our amazing agent, Dan Mandel, who believed in our vision. Our editor, Renee Sedliar, who took a chance on us and made this entire process an amazing experience—thank you. A huge thank you to the entire team at Da Capo and the Perseus Books Group for helping us create this book better than we could have even imagined. We are especially grateful to Lori Hobkirk, Iris Bass, Sandy Chapman, Lissa Warren, and Christine Dore for all their hard work and dedication.

To our experts—chef Jason Brown and trainer extraordinaire Liz Barnet who contributed their time, energy, and amazing skills—we cannot thank you enough!

To the B Nutritious team, both past and present, especially Rachelle LaCroix Mallik and Ying Lam, thank you for all those hours in the kitchen and the office.

We would also like to thank Jennifer Fisherman Ruff, Jamie Rosen, Jacqui Stafford, Brigitte Zeitlin, Andrew James Pierce, Charis West, Diane Foster, and Kristin Collins. And all the early diet testers who gave us such great feedback.

To our families, Hank and Gerry Alpert, David and Mia Alpert, Helen Rodbell, Luke Schlumbrecht, Jennifer and Lee McMillan, Lindsay and Joe Dawson, Kelley Farris and Brett Slocum. Thank you for all your support and encouragement. Todd and Emma — I love you more than you can possibly know.

BIBLIOGRAPHY

Introduction

Boyle, J. P., T. J. Thompson, E. W. Gregg, et al. "Projection of the Year 2050 Burden of Diabetes in the U.S. Adult Population: Dynamic Modeling of Incidence, Mortality, and Prediabetes Prevalence." *Popular Health Metrics* 8 (2010): 29.

Lustig, R. H., L. A. Schmidt, and C. D. Brindis. "Public Health: The Toxic Truth About Sugar." *Nature* 482, no. 7383 (2012): 27–29.

Chapter 3: The Sweet Dilemma

Abou-Donia, M. B., E. El-Masry, A. A. Abdel-Rahman, et al. "Splenda Alters Gut Microflora and Increases Intestinal P-glycoprotein and Cytochrome P-450 in Male Rats." *Journal of Toxicology and Environmental Health, Part A* 71 (2008): 1415–1429.

Ahmed, N. "Advanced Blycation End-Products—Role in Pathology of Diabetic Complications." *Diabetes Research and Clinical Practice* 52 (2005): 673–621.

Avena, N. M., P. Rada, and B. G. Hoebel. "Evidence for Sugar Addiction: Behavioral and Neurochemical Effects of Intermittent, Excessive Sugar Intake." *Neuroscience and Biobehavioral Reviews* 32, no. 1 (2007): 20–39.

Basciano, H., L. Federico, and K. Adeli. "Fructose, Insulin Resistance and Metabolic Dyslipidemia." *Nutrition and Metabolism* 2, no. 1 (2005): 5–19.

Centers for Disease Control and Prevention. "Summary Health Statistics for U.S. Adults: National Health Interview Survey," 2010; updated January 2012. Accessed November 28, 2012. http://www.cdc.gov/nchs/data/series/sr_10/sr10_252.pdf.

Contreras, C. L., and K. Chapman-Novakofski. "Dietary Advanced Glycation End Products and Aging." *Nutrients* 2 (2010): 1247–1265.

Davidson, T. L., A. A. Martin, K. Clark, et al. "Intake of High-Intensity Sweeteners Alters the Ability of Sweet Taste to Signal Caloric Consequences: Implications for the Learned Control of Energy and Body Weight Regulation." *The Quarterly Journal of Experimental Psychology* 64, no. 7 (2011): 1430–1441.

Ford, E.S., C. Li, and G. Zhao. "Prevalence and Correlates of Metabolic Syndrome Based on a Harmonious Definition Among Adults in the US." *Journal of Diabetes* 2, no. 3 (2010): 180–193.

Howard, B. V., and J. Wylie-Rosett. "Sugar and Cardiovascular Disease." *American Heart Association Journal* 106 (2002): 523–527.

Liu, S, W. C. Willett, M. J. Stampfer, et al. "A Prospective Study of Dietary Glycemic Load, Carbohydrate Intake, and Risk of Coronary Heart Disease in US Women." *American Journal of Clinical Nutrition* 71 (2000): 1455–1461.

Livingston, E. H., and J. W. Zylke. "Progress in Obesity Research: Reasons for Optimism." *Journal of the American Medical Association* 308, no. 11 (2012): 1162–1164.

Mozumdar, A., and G. Liguori. "Persistent Increase of the Prevalence of Metabolic Syndrome Among U.S. Adults: NHANES III to NHANES 1999–2006." *Diabetes Care* 43, no. 1 (2011): 216–219.

Pollock, N. K., V. Bundy, W. Kanto, et al. "Greater Fructose Consumption Is Associated with Cardiometabolic Risk Markers and Visceral Adiposity in Adolescents." *Journal of Nutrition* 142, no. 2 (2012): 251–257.

Semba, R. D., E. J. Nicklett, and L. Ferrucci. "Does Accumulation of Advanced Glycation End Products Contribute to Aging Phenotype?" *Journals of Gerontology, Series A: Biological and Medical Sciences* 65A, no 9 (2010): 963–975.

Tappy, L., and K. A. Lê. "Metabolic Effects of Fructose and the Worldwide Increase in Obesity." *Physiological Reviews* 90 (2010): 23–46.

United States Department of Agriculture. "Profiling Food Consumption in America." Accessed November 28, 2012. http://www.usda.gov/factbook/chapter2.pdf.

Yilmaz, Y. "Fructose in Non-Alcoholic Fatty Liver Disease" (review article). *Alimentary Pharmacology and Therapeutics* 35 (2012): 1135–44.

Chapter 4: Sugar: Not So Sweet for Your Skin, Either

Basta, G. "Receptor for Advanced Glycation End-Products and Atherosclerosis: From Basic Mechanisms to Clinical Implications." *Atherosclerosis* 196 (2008): 9–21.

Berra, B., and A. M. Rizzo. "Glycemic Index, Glycemic Load: New Evidence for a Link with Acne." *Journal of the American College of Nutrition* 28, no. 4 (2009): 450S–454S.

Bowe, W.P., S.S. Joshi, A. R. Shalita. "Diet and Acne." *Journal of American Academy of Dermatology* 63 no.1 (2010): 123–141.

Corstjens J., D. Dicanio , N. Muizzuddin, et al. "Glycation associated skin autofluorescence and skin elasticity are related to chronological age and body mass index of healthy subjects." *Experimental Gerontology* 43 (2008): 663–667.

Danby, F. W. "Nutrition and Aging Skin: Sugar and Glycation." *Clinical Dermatology* 28 (2010): 409–411.

Gkogkolou, P., M. Böhm. "Advanced Glycation End Products: Key Players in Skin Aging?" *Dermato-Endocrinology* 4 no. 3 (2012): 259–270.

Jeanmarie, C., L. Danoux, G. Pauly. Glycation during human dermal intrinsic and actinic ageing: an in vivo and in vitro model study. *British Journal of Dermatology* 145 (2001): 10–18.

Noordam, R., D. A. Gunn, C. C. Tomlin, et al. "High Serum Glucose Levels Are Associated with a Higher Perceived Age." *Age: Journal of the American Aging Association* 35, no.1 (2011): 189–195.

O'Brien J, P. A.Morrisey. "Nutritional and toxicological aspects of the Maillard Browning reaction in foods." *Critical Reviews in Food Science and Nutrition* 28 (1989): 211–248.

Ohshima, H., M. Oyobikawa, A. Tada, et al. Melanin and facial skin fluorescence as markers of yellowish discoloration with aging. *Skin Research and Technology* 15 (2009): 496–502.

Semba, R. D., E. J. Nicklett, and L. Ferrucci. "Does Accumulation of Advanced Glycation End Products Contribute to the Aging Phenotype?" *Journals of Gerontology, Series A: Biological and Medical Sciences* 65A, no. 9 (2010): 963–975.

Ubach E., J. W. Lentz. "Carbohydrate metabolism and skin." *Archives of Dermatology and Syphilogy* 52 (1945): 301–316.

Ulrich, P., and A. Cerami. "Protein Glycation, Diabetes, and Aging." *Recent Progress in Hormone Research* 56 (2001): 1–21.

Yamauchi M, Prisayanh P, Haque Z. et al. "Collagen cross-linking in sun-exposed and unexposed sites of aged human skin." *Journal of Investigative Dermatology* 97 (1991): 938–941.

Chapter 5: What to Eat

Albert, C. M., C. H. Hennekens, C. J. O'Donnell, et al. "Fish Consumption and Risk of Sudden Cardiac Death." *Journal of the American Medical Association* 279, no. 1 (1998): 23–28.

Allard, J. S., J. A. Baur, K. G. Becker, et al. "Resveratrol Improves Health and Survival of Mice on a High-Calorie Diet." *Nature* 444, no. 7117 (2006): 337–342.

Assuncao, M. L., H. S. Ferreira, A. F. dos Santos, et al. "Effects of Dietary Coconut Oil on the Biochemical and Anthropometric Profiles of Women Presenting Abdominal Obesity." *Lipids* 44, no. 7 (2009): 593–601.

Barger, J. L., T. Kayo, J. M. Vann, et al. "A Low Dose of Dietary Resveratrol Partially Mimics Caloric Restriction and Retards Aging Parameters in Mice." *PLOS ONE* 3, no. 6 (2008): e2264. doi: 10.1371/journal.pone.0002264.

Carter, P., L. J. Gray, J. Troughton, et al. "Fruit and Vegetable Intake and Incidence of Type 2 Diabetes Mellitus: Systematic Review and Meta-Analysis." *British Medical Journal* 341 (2010): c4229.

Chai, S. C., S. Hooshmand, R. L. Saadat, et al. "Daily Apple Versus Dried Plum: Impact on Cardiovascular Disease Risk Factors in Postmenopausal Women." *Journal of the Academy of Nutrition and Dietetics* 112, no. 8 (2012): 1158–1168.

Conceição de Oliveira, M, R. Sichieri, and A. Sanchez Moura. "Weight Loss Associated with a Daily Intake of Three Apples or Three Pears Among Overweight Women." *Nutrition* 19, no. 3 (2003): 253–256.

Dearlove, R. P, P. Greenspan, D. K. Hartie, et al. "Inhibition of Protein Glycation by Extracts of Culinary Herbs and Spices." *Journal of Medicinal Food* 11, no. 2 (2008): 275–281.

Fujioka, K., F. Greenway, J. Sheard, et al. "The Effects of Grapefruit on Weight and Insulin Resistance: Relationship to the Metabolic Syndrome." *Journal of Medicinal Food* 9, no. 1 (2006): 49–54.

Golomb, B. A., S. Koperski, and H. L. White. "Association Between More Frequent Chocolate Consumption and Lower Body Mass Index." *Archives of Internal Medicine* 172, no. 6 (2012): 519–521.

Herder, C. "Tea Consumption and Incidence of Type 2 Diabetes in Europe: The Epic-Interact Case-Cohort Study." *PLOS ONE* 7, no. 5 (2012): e36910.

Josic, J., A. T. Olsson, J. Wickeberg, et al. "Does Green Tea Affect Postprandial Glucose, Insulin and Satiety in Healthy Subjects: A Randomized Controlled Trial." *Nutrition Journal* 9 (2010): 63.

Kendall, C. W., A. R. Josse, A. Esfahani, et al. "The Impact of Pistachio Intake Alone or in Combination with High-Carbohydrate Foods on Post-Prandial Glycemia." *European Journal of Clinical Nutrition* 65, no. 6 (2011): 696–702.

Khan, A., M. Safdar, M. M. A. Khan, et al. "Cinnamon Improves Glucose and Lipids of People with Type 2 Diabetes." *Diabetes Care* 26, no. 12 (2003): 3215–18.

Nagao, T., Y. Komine, S. Soga, et al. "Ingestion of a Tea Rich in Catechins Leads to a Reduction in Body Fat and Malondialdehyde-Modified LDL in Men." *American Journal of Clinical Nutrition* 81, no. 1 (2005): 122–129.

Norris, L. E., A. L. Collene, M. L. Asp, et al. "Comparison of Dietary Conjugated Linoleic Acid with Safflower Oil on Body Composition in Obese Postmenopausal Women with Type 2 Diabetes Mellitus." *American Journal of Clinical Nutrition* 90, no. 3 (2009): 468–476.

Rasmussen, B. M., B. Vessby, M. Uusitupa, et al. "Effects of Dietary Saturated, Monounsaturated, and N-3 Fatty Acids on Blood Pressure in Healthy Subjects." *American Journal of Clinical Nutrition* 83, no. 2 (2005): 221–226.

Rosell, M., N. N. Hakansson, A. Wolk. "Association Between Dairy Food Consumption and Weight Change Over 9 Y in 19,352 Perimenopausal Women." *American Journal of Clinical Nutrition* 84, no. 6 (2006): 1481–1488.

Roussel, R., L. Fezeu, N. Bouby, et al. "Low Water Intake and Risk for New-Onset Hyperglycemia." *Diabetes Care* 34, no. 12 (2011): 2551–2554.

ScienceDaily. "Buckwheat May Be Beneficial for Managing Diabetes." *ScienceDaily.* American Chemical Society (2003). Accessed December 5, 2011. http://www.sciencedaily.com/releases/2003/11/031118072746.htm#.

Shai, I., D. Schwarzfuchs, Y. Henkin, et al. "Weight Loss with a Low-Carbohydrate, Mediterranean, or Low-Fat Diet." *New England Journal of Medicine* 359, no. 3 (2008): 229–241.

Steinmetz, K. A., and J. D. Potter. "Vegetables, Fruit, and Cancer Prevention: A Review." *Journal of the American Dietetic Association* 96, no. 10 (1996): 1027–1039.

Turner, N., K. Hariharan, J. TidAng, et al. "Enhancement of Muscle Mitochondrial Oxidative Capacity and Alterations in Insulin Action Are Lipid Species Dependent." *Diabetes* 58, no. 11 (2009): 2547–2554.

Wedick, N. M., A. Pan, A. Cassidy, et al. "Dietary Flavonoid Intakes and Risk of Type 2 Diabetes in US Men and Women." *American Journal of Clinical Nutrition* 95, no. 4 (2012): 925–933.

Zomer, E., A. Owen, D. J. Magliano, et al. "The Effectiveness and Cost Effectiveness of Dark Chocolate Consumption As Prevention Therapy in People at High Risk of Cardiovascular Disease: Best Case Scenario Analysis Using a Markov Model." *British Medical Journal* (2012): 344.

Chapter 6: What *Not* to Eat

Duffey, K. J., L. M. Steffen, L. Van Horn, et al. "Dietary Patterns Matter: Diet Beverages and Cardiometabolic Risks in the Longitudinal Coronary Artery Risk Development in Young Adults (CARDIA) Study." *American Journal of Clinical Nutrition* 95, no. 4 (2012): 909–915.

Hu, E. A., A. Pan, V. Malik, et al. "White Rice Consumption and Risk of Type 2 Diabetes: Meta-Analysis and Systematic Review." *British Medical Journal* 344 (2012): e1454.

Nettleton, J. A., P. L. Lutsey, Y. Wang, et al. "Diet Soda Intake and Risk of Incident Metabolic Syndrome and Type 2 Diabetes in the Multi-Ethnic Study of Atherosclerosis
(MESA)." *Diabetes Care* 32, no. 4 (2009): 688–694.

Chapter 7: How to Eat

Mekary, R. A., E. Giovannucci, W. C. Willett, et al. "Eating Patterns and Type 2 Dia-
betes Risk in Men: Breakfast Omission, Eating Frequency, and Snacking." *American
Journal of Clinical Nutrition* (2012). doi:10.3945/ajcn.111.028209.
Ostman, E., Y. Granfeldt, L. Persson, et al. "Vinegar Supplementation Lowers Glucose
and Insulin Responses and Increases Satiety After a Bread Meal in Healthy Subjects."
European Journal of Clinical Nutrition 59, no. 9 (2005): 983–988.

Chapter 9: Your Dermal Detox

Babizhayev, M. A., A. I. Deyev, E. L. Savel'yeva, et al. "Skin Beautification with Oral
Non-Hydrolized Versions of Carnosine and Carcinine: Effective Therapeutic Man-
agement and Cosmetic Skincare Solutions Against Oxidative Glycation and Free-Rad-
ical Production As a Causal Mechanism of Diabetic Complications and Skin Aging."
Journal of Dermatological Treatment 5 (2011): 345–384.
Beitner J. Randomized, placebo-controlled, double blind study on the clinical efficacy of
a cream containing 5% alpha-lipoic acid related to photoageing of facial skin. *British
Journal of Dermatology* 149, no.4 (2003): 841–849.
Dearlove, R. P., P. Greenspan, and D. K. Hartle, et al. "Inhibition of Protein Glycation by
Extracts of Culinary Herbs and Spices." *Journal of Medicinal Food* 11 (2008): 275–281.
Draelos, Z. D., M. S. Yatskayer, M. S. Raab, et al. "An Evaluation of the Effect of a Top-
ical Product Containing C-xyloside and Blueberry Extract on the Appearance of Type
II Diabetic Skin." *Journal of Cosmetic Dermatology.* 8 (2009): 147–151.
Farris P. K. "Innovative Cosmeceuticals: Sirtuin Activators and Anti-glycation Com-
pounds." *Seminars in Cutaneous Medicine and Surgery* 30 (2011): 163–166.
Heng, M. C. "Curcumin Targeted Signaling Pathways: Basis for Anti-Photoaging And
Anti- Carcinogenic Therapy." *International Journal of Dermatology* 49 (2010): 608–622.
Peng, X., J. Ma, F. Chen, et al. "Naturally Occurring Inhibitors Against the Formation of
Advanced Glycation End-Products." *Food & Function* 2 (2001): 289–301.
Rout, S. R. Banerjee. "Free Radical Scavenging, anti-glycation and tyrosinase inhibition
properties of a polysaccharide fraction isolated from the rind of Punica granatum."
Bioresource Technology 98 no. 16 (2007): 3159–3163.
Sang, S. X., Shao, N. Bai, C.Y. Lo, et al. "Tea Polyphenol (-)-epigallocatechin-3-gallate:
A New Trapping agent of Reactive Dicarbonyl Species. *Chemical Research in Toxicol-
ogy* 12 (2007): 1862–1870.
Senevirathne, M., and S. K. Kim. "Brown Algae–Derived Compounds as Potential Cos-
meceuticals. " In *Marine Based Cosmeceuticals: Trends and Prospects.* CRC Press (Tay-
lor & Francis Group), 2012: 179–189.
Yuan, J. P., J. Peng, K. Yin, et al. "Potential Health-Promoting Effects of Astaxanthin: A
High-Value Carotenoid Mostly from Microalgae." *Molecular Nutrition & Food Research.*
55 (2001): 150–165.

Chapter 10: The Sugar-Exercise Connection

Jensen, J., P. I. Rustad, A. J. Kolnes, et al. "The Role of Skeletal Muscle Glycogen Breakdown for Regulation of Insulin Sensitivity by Exercise." *Frontiers in Physiology* (2011): 2.

Little, J. P., J. B. Gillen, M. E. Percival, et al. "Low-Volume High-Intensity Interval Training Reduces Hyperglycemia and Increases Muscle Mitochondrial Capacity in Patients with Type 2 Diabetes." *Journal of Applied Physiology* 111 (2001): 1554–1560.

Teixeira-Lemos, E., S. Nunes, F. Teixeira, et al. "Regular Physical Exercise Training Assists in Preventing Type 2 Diabetes Development: Focus on Its Antioxidant and Anti-Inflammatory Properties." *Cardiovascular Diabetology* 10 (2001): 12–27.

Van Dijk, J. W., R. J. Manders, K. Tummers, et al. "Both Resistance and Endurance Type Exercise Reduce the Prevalence of Hyperglycaemia in Individuals with Impaired Glucose Tolerance and in Insulin-Treated and Non-Insulin Treated Type 2 Diabetic Patients." *Diabetologia* 55, no. 5 (2012): 1273–1282.

RECIPE INDEX

INDEX